Positive Birth in a Modern World

FINDING THE BALANCE BETWEEN THE LAW OF NATURE AND TECHNOLOGY

KAREN WILMOT

The Virtual Midwife

First Printing, 2018

The Virtual Midwife Press

www.thevirtualmidwife.com

Table of Contents

Foreword

by Lisa Ferland

Mothers everywhere must deal with the stressful uncertainty that comes with pregnancy and giving birth. The unknowns stretch before you as your belly grows and hides the view of your toes, and you can find yourself drowning in uncertainty.

Giving birth in a foreign country, in a foreign language, surrounded by strangers is probably not something you ever thought you'd experience. So much of pregnancy and birth are outside of our control, and if you're anything like me, you have picked up this book because you want to prepare and be as knowledgeable about what might happen to you as possible.

No two births are ever alike and what your friends "back home" experience during their births will be radically different from what you will experience.

As you seek out advice and listen to stories from women who have given birth (both domestically and abroad) before, remember that your experience is yours and yours alone. How you prepare for and react to what happens throughout your pregnancy and birth will shape your memories of this incredibly vulnerable yet empowering time in your life.

After speaking with hundreds of women about their birthing experiences abroad, one crucial thread weaves its way throughout all of their stories. They all remember their birth experiences with heartwrenching all-encompassing love – such a huge love that transforms even the most difficult moments into something beautiful.

You will experience the full spectrum of emotions: anxiety, love, hopelessness, optimism, and fulfilment. This wild hormonal-driven roller coaster ride of emotions is normal – lucky us, right? Creating life generates conflicting and bittersweet emotions, so be forgiving of yourself and others.

I've felt the strain of straddling multiple countries at once – the old and the new – and have felt my cultural identity go into meltdown and reform as my babies turned into toddlers. What I once thought was important in my old life no longer mattered in my new world.

I gave birth in the super medicalised approach in the United States and underwent ultrasound scans and urine analyses at every monthly appointment. I've also given birth in Sweden where the midwife told me she'd see me in five months for my next appointment after entering my name and address into the system. With the radical change of healthcare approaches, I had so many questions that nobody could answer.

Did it really matter that I wasn't going to be weighed every four weeks? Would my Swedish midwife who felt my belly with her hands and refused ultrasound scans miss something that a US midwife would have discovered? And more importantly, could I change the local system even if I wanted to? I'll never know, and neither will you.

It is naive of me to suggest that you not compare and contrast at all, because you will. In pregnancy, you will search for something familiar in which to anchor your drifting boat.

Prepare for your birth like you would any other life-altering moment. There will always be a before and an after. Giving birth creates a mini prime meridian in your life by which you mark time. Giving birth abroad undoubtedly adds a few layers of complexity, but they aren't anything that you cannot handle.

Take control of the aspects that are within your control and let go of those that are not. You cannot control for so many elements related to pregnancy and birth, but you can control your breathing, your reactions to the unexpected, and your mental preparation.

By reading this book, you have already taken some control of the elements that are within your sphere of influence. Bringing life into this world without the support from your family is one of the most challenging and stressful things you'll ever have to do, but with this guide and the support of your peers, you will find that you can do incredible things.

I wish you the best as you embrace the beginning of one of the most beautiful chapters in your life.

Lisa Ferland
Author of *Knocked Up Abroad*

Introduction

My story

It is said that one's life purpose is intimately tied to one's life lesson, and for me that has involved a deep and troubling irony. I recall thinking about having babies from a very young age. I recall my own mom finding me under the dining room table drinking milk (which I hated) and trying to breastfeed my doll. I recall visiting neighbours with babies to touch and hold and stare at them. It seems I had this baby radar thing even then; if there was a new baby in town, I would find it. In retrospect, I must have driven those women crazy, but I couldn't help myself. Babies (and the colour pink) were my favourite thing.

My mother was a midwife and I was so proud of her. She always seemed to come home from work glowing with joy and she would tell me about the babies that had been born into her hands. Her face would light up and she would become animated when she shared these stories with my father and I could see how proud he was of her too. I would tell anyone who would listen that she had delivered 100 babies. I am sure it was many more than that, but 100 babies seemed so mysteriously appealing to me and all I wanted when I grew up was to be a midwife and to have 100 babies of my own.

But my mother got cancer at the age of 35 and within two years, despite an above-knee amputation and aggressive chemotherapy, she died peacefully in our home, surrounded by our extended family. I don't remember much about the two years leading up to her death except for vivid memories of a family road trip that we took in our well-loved family Volkswagon station wagon, strangely named Jezabel. My brother and I were taken out of school and we travelled the length and breadth of South Africa, sleeping in the car when we were not staying with friends or family. I remember the celebration when the odometer clicked over to indicate that Jezabel had done 100 000 km. Mom was driving and dad cracked open a bottle of champagne, the cork soaring out of the car window and disappearing into the brown scrub of the old Transvaal Lowveld. We stopped on the side of the road and had a picnic of cold pork sausages and boiled eggs, my brother and I drinking sweet coffee from a flask and my parents touching their plastic mugs of champagne together in a toast. They had not hidden the details of her illness from us, but even so, they framed the trip as a celebration, as parents who wanted to protect their children from the harsh realities of life do. But I caught a moment between them that day. As their plastic mugs touched and they looked at us and then into each other's eyes, their joy dissolved into sadness at the reality of our situation. We all felt it and a strange silence descended upon us. Mom reached her arms out, embracing all of us with a love that was so warm and overwhelming that I can still feel it if I close my eyes and allow myself too. At 8, I was still way too young to grasp the implications of death or the finality of it. All I felt was my mother's deep and unconditional love.

This feeling has driven me all of my life. It has shaped who I am, what I do and the way that I do it. But the circumstances of my life changed when my mother got cancer. Our family dynamic changed when she died and I changed from the carefree happy child who visited all the neighbours to a confused and slightly rebellious teenager. My rebellion was exacerbated when my father remarried a few years later and my image of home and family was tainted.

I left home when I was 17 and stayed true to my dream of studying nursing and midwifery. I completed my training holding onto my vision of setting up an independent practice one day. Although I now have my practice, I am not sure how I would have felt if someone had given me a glimpse into the future and shown me the ironic twist of my life path - for though I would bring countless babies into the world I would never have children of my own.

I never chose not to have children and always assumed that I would have them. But life had other ideas, and I watched the window of opportunity closing as the years flew by and I recognised that it might never happen. I followed my heart and travelled the world, using my nursing and midwifery experience to land jobs in adventurous locations and ultimately leading me to the expat life that I now live so comfortably.

There was a time in my late 30s when I stepped away from my work as a midwife. It did not seem right that I felt so empty and bereft in the face of such happiness and celebration. It felt as if I gave my heart to every mother whose baby I delivered as I handed her baby to her. The magnitude of their happiness did not even begin to resemble the depth of my sadness. I started to feel like a fraud being with women in labour when I had never experienced it myself, ignoring the fact that most of the obstetricians I worked with were men who had never done it either or that the doctors who looked after my mother had never experienced cancer. I grieved for more than the loss of my dream of becoming a mother. I grieved for the loss of family, my family and my mother. I can now admit that I grieved for eight years during which time I did a lot of deep searching. One of my spiritual teachers encouraged me to explore the meaning of a mother. It was through this process, slow and often painful, that I discovered and embraced the mother that I already was. I dipped my toes hesitantly back into the birth world, but with a new perspective. I realised that my ability lay in mothering the mother and that my capacity to love was limitless. I found my voice and acknowledged my gift.

This realisation and the vulnerability that allowed me to embrace my new role has transformed my life and my practice and allowed me to achieve the vision that I had as a child. I have my 100 babies, in fact I have more than a 1 000 now. They are not my babies, but I have been so intimately involved in their birth, that they carry a piece of my heart, and I carry them in mine. Those babies fill my heart to overflowing. They have taught me so much about myself, my ability, my resilience, my strength, my weakness, my capacity to give and receive and mostly, about the mother that I am.

Not having children of my own has driven me to never stop learning, never stop questioning and never to be judgemental. I am not able to project my own experience onto yours and I bring the wisdom of every birth I have attended into my work. It has given me the freedom to continue to travel and to be a pioneer of change in the Middle East where I spent 14 years as an expat and was instrumental in creating the first mother and baby wellness centre in the Gulf region in 2016.

It was during this time, while working as an independent midwife in the community, that I met Jason and Rebecca.

The first time I saw Rebecca, she was sitting on a deck chair in the middle of a large living room, sobbing quietly. There was no other furniture whatsoever and my footsteps echoed loudly on the cold marble floors as I entered the empty space. Jason unfolded another deck chair, which he placed directly in front of Rebecca, motioning for me to take a seat. Then he ducked back into the doorway, looking nervous. I sat down quietly and placed my hands on Rebecca's knees. She was clutching soggy tissues in both hands and still the tears ran down her cheeks.

I sat quietly for at least 20 minutes feeling her confusion, sadness and fear before she finally looked up and spoke. I was acutely aware of Jason behind me in the doorway, seeing his future flashing before his eyes and knowing how crucial this moment was. They were newly married and had just arrived in Oman for their first expat assignment. This was his dream job and they had packed up life as they knew it in New Zealand to save a nest egg for their future. While the pregnancy was very much wanted, it was sooner than expected. A day after they arrived sooner. Their furniture was still en-route and they were still acutely aware of the strong pull of the ties to family and friends.

Rebecca was adamant that they should return immediately. She knew nobody. This was not her home. She did not want to have a baby in these circumstances. This was not how she imagined it. Jason wanted to make it work, to give it time, to at least give it a try.

I don't recall exactly what I said to Rebecca that day, but I know that it was enough to stop her from getting on the next plane home. I invited her to my prenatal yoga classes and three weeks later she tiptoed shyly into class. What followed is what I have outlined in this book, the book I wish I had been able to give Rebecca that day and the book she wished she had had. This is your go-to manual for having a baby abroad, but will be just as helpful if you are in the comfort of your own home country. The references to being abroad will open your mind to possibilities that you may not previously have considered. I encourage you to join my online community so that you can get access to the information that I am constantly creating and updating in my resources library.

FINDING OUT YOU ARE PREGNANT

Whether your pregnancy is planned or not, the moment you see the little blue line is life changing. A thousand thoughts flash through your mind, peppered with images of cuddly babies, happy families and buckets of dirty diapers. It is a rollercoaster of emotion, not least because you are already under the influence of pregnancy hormones. If you are living abroad, away from your home country and the comfort and ease of a medical system you understand, it may well catapult you into a state of panic. This book is just for you. I will virtually take your hand and guide you step by step through the various stages of your pregnancy, signposting the decisions you may need to make and highlighting the options. But, before we start, let's put this all into perspective:

What will be different about having your baby if you are not in your home country?

• You will not have your close family members and friends nearby during memorable and sometimes vulnerable moments.
• You will be thrown into a foreign healthcare system, possibly with foreign doctors, nurses and midwives.
• The language may be different to your own and you will have to navigate appointments and doctor's visits differently.
• You will need to learn a new way of listening, talking and communicating to eliminate things getting lost in translation (or consider having a local to translate for you).
• You will be faced with cultural differences in the way that pregnancy and childbirth are viewed that may not mirror your own.
• You will have to be very clear about what you want and what you need in order to get it.
• The ease of access to baby equipment, gadgets and paraphernalia may be limited, which means shopping online or planning a shopping vacation.
• The ease of access to care providers who "speak your language" or give you the care and attention you so require at this time may be hard to find.

What will be the same, even if you are not in your home country?

• You will want the very best care for you and your baby and you will do whatever you need to do in order to get it.
• You will experience the same highs and lows that come with a normal pregnancy due to hormonal fluctuations, physical changes and life circumstances.
• You will need to have the same tests, examinations and scans you would in your home country, but it may not be as easy to access them, or you may have to request them. You may even be ridiculed for wanting them, given the cultural differences in the way that pregnancy and childbirth are viewed.
• Your pregnancy will progress in the same way that it would were you in your home country and you will experience the same physical changes and discomforts.
• You will face fear of the unknown, which will be compounded by the challenges associated with being in a foreign country. Both will need to be addressed separately and together.
• You will still need to plan and prepare for your birth, but you will be forced to do more research into the available options. This is actually a very good thing.
• You will be overwhelmed by the ease of access to unlimited amounts of information online, which will scare and confuse you.
• You will be faced with many choices and decisions about your pregnancy and birth (like where to give birth, who to have with you and how you will cope with the intensity of the experience).
• You will embark on a journey of deep transformation as you watch your body changing, feeling your baby moving inside you and embracing your new role as a parent.
• You will undergo change, and with change there is ultimately loss. Despite the indescribable joy that comes with having a new baby, it brings some necessary losses in your lifestyle, freedom and some of your income.
• You will need to find someone you can trust to guide and support you through this transformation.

Five things to do if you want your pregnancy to be a positive experience:

1. Don't let fear steal your joy – replace fear with curiosity.
2. Take full responsibility for your health and wellbeing.
3. Connect with like-minded people and new parents in your local community.
4. Research and educate yourself so that you know what to expect.
5. Embrace any differences you might encounter and prepare yourself for cultural misunderstandings.

The chapters of this book cover the seven main questions you will find yourself asking as you prepare yourself for a positive pregnancy experience:
1. Where should my baby be born?
2. How will I monitor the progression of my pregnancy?
3. How will I know what is normal and expected as my body changes during pregnancy?
4. How will I optimise my health and wellness during pregnancy?

5. How can I prepare myself mentally and emotionally for the birth process?
6. How can I prepare myself physically for the birth process and understand what's going to happen as I go into labour?
7. How will I know what common hospital interventions I really need?

By the end of this book you will have the answer to these questions, and much more.

1. Deciding where to give birth

How to decide on the country and the facility in which to give birth

One of the biggest decisions that you will make is deciding where your baby will be born. This includes choosing both the country and the birth facility, for example, home, hospital or birth centre.

Bear in mind that you have time to do this. Right now you are merely doing your homework. Keep an open mind and do not close yourself off to possibilities that you may not previously have considered.

I learned a valuable lesson from a member of the Oman Royal family who I had the pleasure and privilege of working with. She had the means to give birth wherever she chose and, in fact, her family owned one of the private hospitals. However, at the last moment she decided that she wanted to go to the public hospital instead. We arrived in a convoy of Range Rovers at 2 a.m. and while we were ushered through the system slightly more smoothly than usual, she was treated the same as all the other labouring women there. She did not make any fuss when given the oversized and very unflattering hospital gown. She settled into her not so perfect surroundings and just got on with having her baby. Granted, she was transferred to the Royal Suite after birth, where she was able to receive the appropriate VIP treatment, but I was humbled and inspired by her ability to be so flexible and accommodating, given her position and means. Public hospitals are generally very institutional looking. The decor is drab and this one was no different. When I questioned her afterwards about her last-minute decision, she said that she felt more secure at the hospital where her mother had given birth to her and where she knew that there were facilities available in the event of things not going according to plan. Her need for that feeling of security trumped the need to be pampered in luxury. An aesthetically pleasing environment is not the only thing that matters.

Most of the women that I have worked with do not remember what I said to them or the exact words that I used, but they remember that I made them feel safe and secure. The core element of our relationship is trust. Your overall experience relies on many factors, but trust is vital. By the end of this book you should know enough to be able to trust yourself to make decisions, to trust your partner to support you, to find a care provider that you trust, and to choose to have your baby in a place where you trust that your wishes and desires will be respected.

It is quite likely that you have never actually *thought much about what kind of birth you would like to have*. You have definitely wondered how a baby can get out of such a small place and no doubt that has been a scary thought. After all, "that place" is presently associated with pleasure. While the knowledge of how to give birth is inherent in all of us, as women, the recent medicalisation of birth requires a learned knowledge of how to navigate the system and the many choices you will be faced with, and this is what I outline in this book.

You may have heard of a midwife named Ina May Gaskin who is regarded as a pioneer for natural birth, albeit hippy style. Like many people who become known for creating positive change, she never set out to do it. She was just following her heart and doing what she thought was right. In 1977 she published her first book, *Spiritual Midwifery*, which presented pregnancy, childbirth and breastfeeding from a fresh, natural and spiritual perspective, rather than the standard clinical viewpoint. By the early 1990s, it was acknowledged as a classical text on midwifery. She continues to run her midwifery centre, The Farm, in Tennessee and continues to have outstanding birth outcomes with an average C-section rate of less than 2%. Considering that the WHO recommends a C-section rate of 15% and that most hospitals are operating at over 50%, this is phenomenal. While there are many contributing factors, I truly believe that this is directly attributable to her deep belief in and respect for the birthing woman and the power and pleasure of birth.

I bring this up because, in my experience, most women's expectation of birth is that it is dangerous, painful and generally unpleasant. This notion is heightened by the media who love to portray birth as dramatic and life-threatening. Most women I work with start their pregnancy from a place of fear and it takes time and effort to change their mindset to the possibility of birth being a powerfully transformative experience.

Now that you are pregnant yourself, you know that your baby has to come out. While there is an option for an elective C-section which would allow you to choose the date and be fully prepared, you will need to undergo major abdominal surgery which carries risks of its own. Often I have worked with women who have come to me quite certain that they wanted a planned C-section with all the drugs. But the more they learnt and educated themselves, the more open they become to the possibilities of a natural birth with all of its benefits to both mom and baby. Stay open and don't rush to make your decision. It is really important to research all the options available to you, and when you find the one that seems right for you, given your circumstances, to plan your preparation around that.

Very often, in your eagerness to find the right information, you forget to ask the basic question of what feels right for you. It is a bit like knowing that you are hungry but not knowing what you want to eat. You go shopping and fill your trolley, but by the time you get home you still have no idea of what you are going to make, despite having a trolley full of options. However, if you knew you wanted lasagna, you would make sure you had pasta, meat and sauce and you would put them all together to make a lovely meal. If you want lasagna in a foreign country, you might have to look a bit longer and harder to find the right ingredients and you might have to substitute a few brands that may not be available, but you will still be able to make lasagna.

There are several factors that you will need to take into consideration if you choose to have your baby abroad. Let's look at the country considerations first.

LEGAL CONSIDERATIONS

Begin by visiting the embassy or consulate of your home country in your host country and get clear instructions on how to register the birth of your baby and how to get a passport once your baby is born.

Ensure that there are no loopholes that you need to be aware of, or anything extra that you need to do before or after the birth.

In some parts of the world, like the Middle East, you will need your marriage certificate to register the birth of your baby. Get these papers in order and ready so that there is no last-minute panic.

If you are considering a home birth, you will need to find out if it is available in your host country and whether it carries any legal implications.

POLITICAL CONSIDERATIONS

It goes without saying that if there is any form of political unrest or instability, it would be wise to consider returning to your home country.

MEDICAL CONSIDERATIONS

Get a complete list of services provided by your medical insurance company. Then visit the local clinic or hospital in the area and assess the services available for pregnancy care as well as the birth facilities. Remember that your pregnancy (or prenatal) care and the birth facility are usually two different areas in the hospital with different staff or possibly even two different hospitals. Your priority in the beginning of pregnancy is checking the services available for prenatal care.

Assses the overall look and feel of the place, along with standards of hygiene, systems and ability to make yourself heard and understood. Stay open-minded, especially if you are in a country that is very different to your own. Put your expat eyes on and see things as they are, not as you would like them to be. There is still plenty of time to scout around or to make alternative arrangements if you are not happy with what is available.

Use the Routine Tests and Investigations Cheat Sheet (www.thevirtualmidwife.com/resources) as a guideline for your care. Take it with you to the clinic, midwife or doctor that you plan to see and use it to open a discussion about your care plan:

Ask them if they offer all of the tests and investigations. If they have a different schedule, ask them to explain it to you so that you are reassured that it is adequate for your needs. As you read in the foreword of this book, your expectations may be vastly different to the reality, but don't allow that to influence you negatively or make rushed decisions. Different countries have different schedules and ways of doing things - the cheat sheet is your guideline.

Ask if there are any tests or investigations over and above what is outlined in the plan that they recommend and if there are, ask where they are available and when you should get them. Stay in the present moment. While you are using this to plan ahead, make sure that you get the care you need now and that you feel satisfied with the standard of care. You still have plenty of time to plan your birth and to decide on where you will give birth. At this stage you are planning your pregnancy. Wherever possible, take a local translator or friend with you if there is a language difference and be very clear in the way that you ask questions and interpret answers. Do not be afraid to ask the same question in different ways until you are satisfied with the answer. Stay open and friendly. You are not underestimating their ability to provide good healthcare, you are merely making sure that you are comfortable with what is available. Plan any travel, whether it is a short holiday, a babymoon or a trip home to get additional tests, around this initial discussion.

Connect with the local expat community and use social media channels to ask for advice about finding a good prenatal class and a local doula. Join any pregnancy and birth-related local clubs or groups and seek out like-minded couples. Local groups will be your support network, but only if you allow them to be. Being pregnant abroad requires a shift in mindset and it begins right now. I highly recommend seeking out a doula to support you during pregnancy, birth and the fourth trimester. The main role of a doula is to help you feel supported and informed and to guide you to find the best resources. Most doulas are also able to offer childbirth education as part of your preparation for birth which is essential if you want a positive birth experience.

Remember – your care plan for pregnancy is different to your care plan for birth. Most couples prefer to have their baby at the same hospital with the same care provider who has attended to them throughout the pregnancy. While this is usually preferable and allows for continuity of care, it does not have to be this way. Give yourself room to change and move about to get the best care in the right place at the right time.

BIRTH FACILITY CONSIDERATIONS

The day you give birth should be as beautiful and memorable as other milestones in your life and it should involve as much, if not more, planning and preparation so that it is a positive experience for you, your baby and your partner. Your choice of birth place will impact many of the decisions that you will need to make during pregnancy and how you go about preparing yourself. While nothing about childbirth itself has changed, evolving technology will influence the way you view and learn about pregnancy and childbirth. Your mother did not face nearly as many choices in her care. She did not have the array of pain management options or diagnostic technology that is now offered, much like a menu in a restaurant. There is no shortage of information available to you. Your challenge is discerning the information that inspires curiosity rather than fear and using that information in a way that serves you and your partner, guiding you to make informed decisions.

The truth is that you will be giving birth within a system that practises defensive medicine, where birth is treated as a medical emergency rather than a life event. You will be offered interventions that, when used appropriately, can be lifesaving. However, they also hold the potential to be misused within a risk-averse environment that promotes interventions to prevent complications and avoid litigation; as much as for financial gain. This is not to say that you should choose a home birth over a hospital birth. There is no right and wrong here. Rather, it is about being mindful of the implications of your choice and the importance of being physically, mentally and emotionally prepared.

Unassisted home birth

This is not the choice of most women and in many ways is quite radical as you will be giving birth without the support of a midwife, doula or doctor and with no backup in the event of complications. While I support it in the right circumstances with the right preparation, I would not recommend it and have only included it as it is still an option, albeit not for the majority.

Home birth with a midwife

• During pregnancy: All your antenatal care will be done by your midwife and you will only be referred to an obstetrician if you are high risk or present with any complications.
• During birth: Independent midwives have all the equipment required to assist a normal birth and cope with minor complications.
• Pain relief: Midwives are licensed to carry and administer pain relief medication and most have gas and air (Entonox). They will encourage and support you with nonmedical comfort measures. Many of them work together with a doula who is trained to offer nonmedical support. Midwives are trained to recognise when things are not proceeding within the range of what is normal and will make a call to transfer you to hospital in the event of an emergency or complications that cannot be managed within the home setting.

• After birth: Your midwife will continue to do home visits for 2-6 weeks after birth to assist you with feeding and settling into motherhood.

Most midwives work in teams. Unfortunately, not all countries offer midwife-led care and not all countries have independent midwives. Do your research, ask around, and find out as much as you can before making your decision.

Birth centre

This is a home-like facility existing within a healthcare system with a programme of care designed in the wellness model of pregnancy and birth.

• During pregnancy: You will be attended throughout your pregnancy, during birth and after your birth by a midwife who works at the birth centre. You will only be referred to an obstetrician in the event of complications.

• During birth: Your midwife will be with you during the birth and will deliver your baby. The obstetrician will only be called in the event of an emergency.

• Pain relief: All pain relief options are available in birth centres and they will support and encourage nonmedical comfort measures as well. Most birth centres have staff doulas to attend to your comfort throughout your labour. Some birth centres offer epidurals.

• Complications: They have facilities to do emergency C-sections but they do not do elective C-sections. Once again, not all countries have birth centres, so do your research, ask around, and find out as much as you can before making your decision.

• After birth: Most birth centres offer home visits for 2-6 weeks following discharge and you will be well supported by a team of midwives. postnatal doulas and breastfeeding consultants.

Private hospital

• During pregnancy: You will see your obstetrician at their private practice rooms for all your antenatal visits throughout your pregnancy.

• During birth: You will not meet your midwife until you are in labour, at which stage she will look after you throughout labour and only call your obstetrician when you are ready to give birth or in the event of complications.

• Pain relief: All pain relief options, medical and nonmedical, are available. Epidural rates tend to be higher in private hospitals.

• Complications: In the event of serious complications, you may have to be transferred to a larger government hospital, depending on what facilities are available. They are also risk averse due to fear of litigation, so intervention rates are high. You will need to be proactive. I will be teaching you how to use the BRAT questioning technique covered in a later chapter so that you are able to confidently participate in all decision making.

• After birth: Most hospitals do not offer any form of follow-up home care after discharge and you will be left to figure out newborn care on your own. The first weeks at home are intense. I highly recommend hiring a doula who includes postnatal care in her package.

Public/government hospital

During pregnancy: You will be seen in the health clinic for all your antenatal care and may see a different obstetrician every time.

• During birth: You will not meet your midwife until you are in labour. Midwives work in teams and they tend to be very busy without much time for quality one-to-one care. The obstetrician will be called only in the event of complications. Care is less personalised as there are more beds and less staff.

• Pain relief: All pain relief options, medical and nonmedical, are available. Epidurals are not always available.

• Complications: Public and government hospitals usually function as training hospitals so they have facilities and expertise to cope with extreme complications. Public hospitals work according to strict procedures and protocols and there is not much room for individualised care. You will need to be proactive and know how to use the BRAT questioning techniques.

• After birth: Most hospitals do not offer any form of follow-up home care after discharge and you will be left to figure out newborn care on your own. The first weeks at home are intense. I highly recommend hiring a doula who includes postnatal care, unless you have a package with me, in which case it is included.

FINANCIAL CONSIDERATIONS

Expats usually have fairly comprehensive medical insurance policies as part of their relocation package. Bigger multinational companies usually have dedicated clinics in remote areas or they will have a list of recommended doctors. Remember that you are not the first expat to be pregnant in the country or company, so start off by getting a complete list of exactly what is covered by your insurance, what services the company you work for offers and what is available in the country you are in.

Some medical insurance policies will only cover the most basic care and may be prohibitive on prenatal classes and post-natal care. I strongly urge you to put some money aside for these vital services that will give you the reassurance and peace of mind that you seek. Insurance policies cover basic medical expenses and do not see the value in complementary services even in the context of pregnancy and birth, which is essentially a life event. It may seem to be an added extra that you can do without but the value of confidence in your ability to birth your baby and to parent is priceless. Now more than ever you need the reassurance that only a professional can give you. Do not rely on Google for advice and direction as most of what you read will not apply to you or your particular situation. Budget for a good prenatal class, a private midwife or a doula and some dedicated post-natal care.

2. Monitoring your pregnancy

Assessing the health-monitoring options in your host country and understanding the routine tests and investigations you will need

Your next step in deciding whether you should stay in your host country for the pregnancy and birth or return home involves assessing the available health-monitoring services. Remember that even if you decide to stay it is never too late to change your mind at a later stage. Pregnancy is a continuum of care and things are constantly in motion and changing.

Do not make the assumption that your care will be better or the outcome guaranteed by returning to the safety of your home country. You will need to do the same amount of research and planning in your home country. You will need to make many of the same choices. You will be faced with similar decisions throughout your pregnancy.

By choosing to return home, you will have the added burden of having to leave your host country at around 32-34 weeks (depending on your airline). Unless your partner is able to take more than six weeks leave to return home with you, you will be separated for the last precious weeks of pregnancy. You will need to weigh up the benefit of being at home with family and in a known environment with the drawback of being separated from your partner. You need to consider that your partner may miss your birth because birth is unpredictable. While you have an estimated due date, there is every possibility that your baby will arrive two weeks early or one week late. That leaves a three-week window of opportunity to decide on booking your flight before, on or after your due date.

Just to put things into perspective, remember that you will only see your doctor or midwife an average of 12 times (or 12 hrs) in a normal 40-week pregnancy. The rest of the time is up to you to look after yourself. Take full responsibility for your own health and well-being. It seems crazy to spend so much time apart as a couple, especially during such a special time, for the sake of 10 visits to your doctor and the standard, routine tests that are required in a low risk, normal pregnancy.

Once you have taken the time to assess the health services in your area and confirmed the availability of facilities to carry out your routine tests, you can put your energy into nurturing and enjoying your pregnancy and planning ahead to get the best care. Of course, this depends a lot on the country and the health facilities available, but take all these things into consideration before making a hasty decision.

An important factor that will influence your decision to stay or go will be whether you are low risk or high risk.

ARE YOU LOW RISK OR HIGH RISK?

Most women are low risk and this will be confirmed at your first visit and reassessed at every subsequent visit. The tests and investigations in this book are standard for all low-risk cases. You will be described as a low-risk pregnancy unless you have a preexisting condition (before you became pregnant) which would place you as a high-risk pregnancy. You will continue to be low risk for as long as you do not present with any symptoms or conditions that would place you at high risk.

Conditions that would place you at high risk include diabetes, hypertension, arthritis, asthma, cardiac disease, kidney problems, liver disease, previous miscarriage, fertility problems (e.g. you needed IVF in order to become pregnant).

If you are in the high-risk category then you may need tests and investigations over and above what is outlined here, which would be determined by your condition. Ask the right questions to ensure that you are able to get the right tests done at the right time, and do not be afraid to get a second opinion.

The following cheat sheet provides a handy guide to the routine tests and investigations you need to know about. For ease of use, you can download a PDF copy on my website at www.thevirtualmidwife.com/resources.

First trimester

Weeks 6-8: You suspect that you are pregnant and go for a test. Your pregnancy will be confirmed with a beta HCG blood test. The doctor may also do a dating scan to measure the fetus and give you a preliminary EDD or expected due date.

Weeks 10-12: You will have your next visit for more blood tests and an ultrasound.

After this you will be seen approximately every 4 weeks (week 16, 20, 24) until you are 28 weeks. The NT scan is due between week 11-14 and the anomaly scan is due between week 18-21 and your visits will be planned around these scans. At each visit your weight, urine and blood pressure will be checked and this is an opportunity to ask your questions and establish a relationship with your doctor or midwife. As mentioned in the foreword by Lisa Ferland, this routine differs from country to country, so use this cheat sheet as your guideline. Discuss the care plan that is offered in your country with the attending doctor or midwife until you feel happy that it is enough for you.

Second trimester

Around week 28, your doctor may request a GTT or glucose tolerance test if there is a high level of glucose in your urine. This is also a good time to do the 4D scan and get pictures to send home. Hereafter, your doctor or midwife may ask to see you for routine weight, urine and blood pressure checks once per fortnight, starting at 32 weeks. Most airlines do not allow you to fly after 32 weeks so if you are planning to return to your home country for the birth then you will need to take this into consideration towards the end of your second trimester. You will also need to ensure that you have appointments booked in your home country and as far as possible try to maintain continuity of care. Give yourself time to meet and establish a relationship with your care provider, just as you have done to date. Go through the same steps of finding suitable care and ask the same questions. Do not make the automatic assumption that the care is better in your home country, and do the same due diligence.

Third trimester

Your visits will become more regular in the last four weeks of pregnancy, with continued routine weight, urine and blood pressure checks. This is the time to start having more in-depth conversations about your birth choices and making sure that your doctor or midwife is clear about your role in your birth and the extent of your preparation so that they can support you.

MAKING SENSE OF THE TEST RESULTS

1. Routine antenatal blood screening

Complete blood count (CBC) is a panel of tests that evaluate the three types of cells that circulate in the blood:
- White blood cells (WBC) are the cells that fight infection in the body.
- Red blood cells (RBC) are the cells that transport oxygen throughout the body.
- Haemoglobin (Hb) is the amount of the oxygen-carrying protein in the blood.

Normal Hb in non-pregnant women is 12-16 grams per decilitre (g/dl), while in pregnant women it should be in the range of 10-14 g/dl.

It is useful to know your blood group (A, B, AB, or O) in case you need to be given blood at any time during pregnancy or during delivery. You will also find out your Rhesus (Rh) factor, which is expressed as negative or positive (– or +)

If you are Rh– you can carry a baby who is Rh+ (if the baby's father is RH+). However, if a small amount of the baby's Rh+ blood enters your Rh– bloodstream during pregnancy or birth, you may produce antibodies against the Rh+ cells known as anti-D antibodies.

If you are Rh–, your blood will be tested for anti-D antibodies, and depending on the result, you may be recommended to have anti-D injections at 28 and 34 weeks of pregnancy, and again after the birth of the baby. This is quite safe for both you and your baby.

This usually doesn't affect the first pregnancy, but you will be more closely monitored in subsequent pregnancies as your immune response will be greater and you may produce a lot more antibodies.

You may also request a TORCH screen which includes testing for toxoplasmosis. This is relevant if you have close contact with stray cats or even if you have cats as pets. The TORCH screen is not a standard part of the routine antenatal blood screening.

Rubella (German measles): Most of us have built up immunity to rubella and your blood test will indicate the level of immunity.

Syphilis: You need to be tested for this sexually transmitted infection as it can lead to miscarriage and stillbirth if left untreated.

Hepatitis B: This virus can cause serious liver disease, and it may infect your baby if you're a carrier or you're infected during pregnancy. Your baby can be immunized at birth to prevent infection. If you have hepatitis B, you will be referred to a specialist.

Hepatitis C: This virus can cause liver disease and there is a small risk it will pass to your baby if you are infected. It cannot be prevented at present so if you are infected, you will be referred to a specialist and your baby can be tested after it is born.

HIV: HIV can be passed to a baby during pregnancy, at delivery or after birth by breastfeeding. If you are HIV positive, both you and your baby can have treatment and care that reduces the risk of your baby becoming infected.

2. Routine examinations at every visit

Your blood pressure, weight and urine should be checked at every antenatal visit and recorded on your antenatal card. This is not done in all countries but I recommend requesting it if it is not done as a routine as we get a lot of useful information from these three simple procedures.

You should be seated in a comfortable position with your arm (left or right) resting on a stable surface at more or less the level of your heart when you get your blood pressure checked. If you are feeling anxious, take a few slow, deep breaths to calm yourself down as this could affect the reading. The blood pressure cuff is wrapped around the upper arm with the lower edge of the cuff at the level of the inside of your elbow and then inflated manually or via a digital monitor. The cuff will deflate slowly and the reading is expressed as a measurement with two numbers, one number on top and one on the bottom, like a fraction, for example 120/80.

The top number (120) refers to the amount of pressure in your arteries during contraction of your heart muscle; this is called "systolic" pressure. The bottom number (80) refers to your blood pressure when your heart muscle is between beats; this is called "diastolic" pressure. A normal blood pressure reading is below 120/80. High blood pressure is defined as anything above 140/90.

It is normal for your blood pressure to rise and fall throughout pregnancy, but your caregiver will be looking for significant or sudden changes. This is why it is important to have your blood pressure checked at every antenatal appointment.

A sudden or gradual increase in blood pressure after 20 weeks of pregnancy may be a sign of pre-eclampsia, but not always. We always need to look at the big picture of symptoms. The exact cause is not known so there is not anything specific that you can do to prevent it, although if you have high BP when you fall pregnant, you will be monitored more closely.

Excessively low BP in pregnancy can be just as problematic as you will feel continuously tired, weak and sometimes dizzy. It is very important to make sure that you are always well hydrated, eating small regular meals and taking enough rest if you have continuously low BP. It will usually resolve in the second trimester.

To check your urine, you will be asked to collect a small sample of clean, midstream urine in a sterile plastic cup. Chemically prepared testing strips are dipped into your sample of urine to screen for certain indicators. A more in-depth analysis may be done by having your urine sample assessed by a laboratory. A urine dip stick test will indicate if there are abnormal levels of sugar, protein, ketones or bacteria in your urine which would indicate further investigation.

It is normal for your kidneys to leak sugar from your bloodstream into your urine. This is particularly expected if you eat a large meal or drink a really sweet beverage, so sugar in your urine does not mean you are diabetic. You should be tested for gestational diabetes only if consistent levels of sugar (glucose) are detected and/or you feel tired or lethargic, if you are consistently thirsty and if you are losing weight despite being pregnant.

Protein found in your urine indicates a problem in kidney function such as an infection. If protein is found in your urine late in pregnancy, this may be a sign of pre-eclampsia. It would usually be associated with one or more other symptoms, such as raised glucose levels, a higher than normal blood pressure reading and swollen face and extremities.

Ketones occur when your body is breaking down fats instead of carbohydrates for energy. High levels of ketones indicate that you are not getting enough to eat or that you are dehydrated.

Bacteria in your urine is a sign of a urinary tract infection. You should be asked for a second urine sample collected through a catheter or similar sterile procedure before determining the treatment or type of antibiotics needed.

3. Ultrasound scans

These days an ultrasound is one of the first and most basic investigations done in pregnancy. Due to their ease and availability, and very often fear, they are being done far more frequently than what is necessary. Ideally, they should only be done when medically indicated. They are simple and painless. Gel is spread on your abdomen to work as a conductor for the sound waves produced via a transducer. The sound waves bounce off bones and tissue returning back to the transducer to generate black and white images of the fetus and you walk away with a picture record for your fridge (and family!) Scans are used as a diagnostic tool to confirm your pregnancy, identify the location of your placenta, and assess the amniotic fluid level. They are also able to measure your baby to verify dates and growth and assess your baby's position. Variations from the norm such as a multiple pregnancy or ectopic pregnancy will also be confirmed via ultrasound.

The Nuchal Translucency scan (NT scan) is done anytime between week 11-14 to assess the risk of certain birth defects, such as Down syndrome, Edward's syndrome (trisomy 18), trisomy 13 and many other chromosomal abnormalities as well as heart problems.

The screening involves two steps. A blood test checks for levels of pregnancy-associated plasma protein-A (PAPP-A) and human chorionic gonadotropin. The nuchal translucency screening measures your baby's nasal bone as well as the fluid at the back of your baby's neck. The combined result of the blood tests and the ultrasound gives you a sense of your baby's risk. However, it's not a diagnosis. Most women who have an abnormal first-trimester screening go on to have healthy babies.

Whether you get this test is your choice. You may want the test so you can prepare or you may decide that knowing the results wouldn't change anything. You may feel that the test could result in unnecessary stress and invasive testing. However knowing of possible risks would allow for increased monitoring during your pregnancy as well as giving you delivery options (special hospital, pediatric surgeon availability) which would be an important consideration when you are planning your birth as an expat.

If your results are normal, your baby has a low risk of these birth defects. If they're abnormal, your doctor may suggest further tests to rule out problems. These could include ultrasounds or invasive procedures, like CVS or amniocentesis.

Remember that this test cannot diagnose birth defects. It only shows if your baby has a greater risk than average, indicating further testing.

Other names for this test include Nuchal test or integrated screening, so bear this in mind when you are discussing your care to avoid misunderstandings and things getting lost in translation. The triple screen, quad screen, MSAFP and sequential screening are tests that are similar to this test and may be offered in the absence of an NT scan. Once again, an awareness of the variables available will help you with your planning.

The anomaly scan is performed anytime between week 18-21. In some areas, it may be carried out later than 21 weeks. The anomaly scan is offered to everybody, but you don't have to have it if you don't want to. The scan checks for major physical abnormalities in your baby, although it can't pick up every problem. It looks in detail at the baby's bones, heart, brain, spinal cord, face, kidneys and abdomen and more specifically for 11 conditions, some of which are very rare:

* anencephaly
* open spina bifida
* cleft lip
* diaphragmatic hernia
* gastroschisis
* exomphalos
* serious cardiac abnormalities
* bilateral renal agenesis
* lethal skeletal dysplasia
* Edwards' syndrome, or T18
* Patau's syndrome, or T13

There are no known risks to the baby or you from having an ultrasound scan, but it's important to think carefully about whether to have the scan or not. As with the NT scan, getting this test is your choice. You may want the test so you can prepare or you may decide that knowing the results wouldn't change anything. You may feel that the test could result in unnecessary stress and invasive testing. If the scan shows there might be a problem, you may be offered chorionic villus sampling (CVS) or amniocentesis or NIPT (DNA-based non-invasive prenatal testing). Developments in genetic technologies have transformed the world of prenatal testing in the last decade. NIPT can be done as early as 10 weeks of pregnancy and results are usually available within two weeks. There is no risk of miscarriage (as with amniocentesis) and results are 99% accurate. If you're offered further tests, you'll be given more information about the tests so you can decide whether or not you want to have them. If necessary, you'll be referred to a specialist, possibly in another hospital and this may affect your choice of where to give birth.

CHOOSING A CARE PROVIDER

Who will look after you during pregnancy? And who will attend your birth?

The most important aspect of your relationship with your chosen care provider is that you feel comfortable and confident. Like any relationship, this takes time and a bit of effort - but bear in mind that most of the effort will be from you. Many doctors are really not that interested in creating a relationship with you. You are a patient and he/she has a job to do - to make sure that you have a healthy pregnancy and birth. If you are in a country where the language and culture are vastly different to your own, accept that this will take more effort on your part and it is largely up to you to make it work. I recall a lovely couple I worked with who chose a particularly difficult doctor despite her weird bedside manner. They knew that she enjoyed a glass of good red wine so they always took a discreetly wrapped bottle along to their consultations.

"A little gift for you, thought you might enjoy this on your day off," Gus would venture before whipping out a list of questions and engaging her in conversation. He made sure that nothing they wanted to discuss was fobbed off with, "Oh we can chat about that closer to the birth," and would press on until they got the answers they were looking for.

Just as we "click" with some people and not with others, you may feel the same with your doctor. There may be an immediate gut reaction of like/dislike/wariness/ease/confidence. It is important to take note of this feeling because very often your first impression is the lasting impression and most often it is correct. When you are newly pregnant, you want your doctor to share your excitement or at least appear to share in it. It is disappointing when they appear not to.

First impressions are more important than what we think. Without realising it, we form an opinion of a person within the first 21 seconds of meeting them. Only seven percent of what we think of them is based on what they say, while 93% of our judgment is based on nonverbal cues like body language. If it is your first visit and your doctor appears disinterested, it may just be due to lack of sleep and the fact that many of the questions that you have can be answered by your midwife or other healthcare professional, whose job it is to educate and support you throughout pregnancy. Much like I do.

Often I speak with women who are disillusioned with their doctors because they do not take the time to speak to them about diet and how to take care of themselves, especially in the first trimester, when excitement is high and they want to make sure they don't miss anything. The harsh reality is that it is not really up to the doctor to tell you this. Their main function in early pregnancy is to assess any inherent risk factors and if you are essentially low risk then it is a normal, healthy pregnancy.

Doctors are trained in pathophysiology. "Patho" relates to disease, dysfunction and abnormality. They are trained to know the difference between the normal and the abnormal and to prevent or treat the abnormal. Their focus is on the pathophysiology because if everything is normal, they are not needed. Pregnancy is a normal physiological process.

THINGS TO THINK ABOUT WHEN CHOOSING YOUR DOCTOR OR CARE PROVIDER

Ask yourself these five questions when choosing a doctor or care provider:

1. What do you expect from your doctor/care provider in a consultation? (For example, mood, personality, demeanour, professionalism, expertise, knowledge, communication, proactive or reactive, guidance, reassurance, and information.) Don't limit yourself. This is an important consideration.

2. What, in your opinion, is the role of the doctor/care provider in YOUR pregnancy? For example, to guide, inform, rule out risk factors, find risk factors, refer, reassure and pamper.

3. What are YOUR beliefs about pregnancy and birth and does your doctor/care provider share your beliefs? How do you know this? How will you discuss this?

4. Are you afraid to change doctor/care provider for fear of hurting their feelings? Is this a business or a personal relationship?

5. Do you trust your gut feeling? How important is trusting your gut feeling in your decision-making process?

I encourage you to answer these questions before your first visit so that you have a clear idea of what it is that you are looking for and your expectations. After your visit, take some time to complete the following five questions to see if your needs were met. If necessary, come back and repeat this exercise again. You may find that your answers change as your pregnancy progresses.

After you have met with your doctor or care provider, ask these five questions:

1. Did you doctor/care provider acknowledge you, address you by your name and give you satisfactory answers to your concerns? How important is this to you?

2. If you have fears surrounding pregnancy and birth, did your doctor/care provider do or say anything to alleviate those fears or refer you to someone to talk to?

3. Did your doctor/care provider say or do anything that increased your fears? Was the focus on risk or safety?

4. Does your doctor/care provider seem to share your beliefs about pregnancy and birth and do they respect your choices?

5. What was your initial gut feeling?

I encourage you to refer back to your answers after each doctor's visit and see if your needs are being met. You might be guided to change your care provider or seek a second opinion. Knowing what you want and what you expect from your doctor or care provider is key to getting what you want. It will also help you manage your expectations and let you know when to seek additional care and assistance.

The following cheat sheet provides a handy guide to all the questions you should ask about your doctor or care provider. You can download a PDF copy on my website at www.thevirtualmidwife.com/resources.

CHOOSING YOUR DOCTOR CHEAT SHEET

Credentials

Is your doctor certified and, if so, by whom?
Where does your doctor attend births (what hospitals and other facilities)?
If your doctor provides home birth services, what systems are in place for transfer if it is necessary?

Practices

Does your doctor have policies for eating and drinking during labour?
Does your doctor have any restrictions on positions during labour and birth?
Does your doctor offer or recommend complementary therapies and, if so, what are they and are there any limitations on their use?
What methods of pain relief do they typically recommend and use?

Statistics

How much time is a typical antenatal appointment and what can you expect?
What is the protocol for induction and what is the induction rate?
What is the C-section rate at the hospital and why are most C-sections performed?
What percentage of woman have an episiotomy? Is it routine practice?

General

Does your doctor work in a group and, if so, does the rest of the team share the same practices?
What does the attitude towards a natural and holistic birth seem to be?
Does your doctor appear to trust the birth process? Is he or she risk averse?
Did you feel patronised or uncomfortable with any of the answers?

In every interaction that you have with your care provider, the questions and answers should be a two-way process. You both need information from each other to ensure the best outcomes for everyone concerned. You are not questioning their ability or experience but trying to deepen your own understanding so that you can make the best decision based on their answers and with the benefit of their insight and expertise. You are merely requesting that they explain their thought processes and discuss various options.

It is important to know how to frame and pose your questions so that you can get the answers that you are seeking without seeming confrontational. If you are in a country with a different language to your own, do a bit of research and learn the words that may be used or consider taking a translator with you to appointments so that you can be sure you are able to ask effective questions and understand the answers - making sure that nothing is lost in translation.

During routine check-ups

Most couples I know expect the doctor to guide the consultation and give them lots of information and that warm fuzzy feeling of being seen and heard. They wait for 45 minutes, see the doctor for 5 minutes and walk out thinking "is that it?" There are two different perspectives to consider. From your point of view, you only have one doctor and you would like to feel as if the doctor you have chosen values and regards you as highly as you do them. From the doctor's point of view, you are one of possibly 15 patients they will see that day. Your symptoms are the same. Your questions are the same. Your fears and anxieties are the same. Most of the time they are more concerned about the medical perspective of your pregnancy than the personal and emotional aspect. While this is good, it does not make for warm, fuzzy feelings. This does not mean that you should change to another doctor (although it would be good to get both), but it will help if you have an idea of what to expect in a consultation and what questions to ask.

This is a bit like when I get my car serviced. I know nothing about cars so I expect the mechanic to tell me if anything is wrong or needs doing. If they don't tell me, I don't know and I don't know enough about it to ask the appropriate questions because I don't know what I don't know. And neither do you when it comes to your care during pregnancy.

Questions to ask during consultations:

• Do you offer all the standard tests and treatments at this hospital/clinic? (Use the Routine Tests and Investigations Cheat Sheet as your guide.)
• Are my pregnancy symptoms normal for the stage of pregnancy that I am at?
• Do I carry any high-risk factors in this pregnancy? (This will be re-assessed at every visit.)
• What should I do if I experience any spotting?
• If I have any risk factors, is this facility capable of handling them appropriately?
• When would you recommend that I see you again?
• What will you do at our next consultation?
• When is my next blood test/scan/routine visit scheduled and what will you be checking for?
• Are there any tests outside of the standard, routine tests that you recommend?
• Is there anything specific I should be doing or watching out for at this stage of my pregnancy?
• Is there anything I need to avoid doing or eating at this stage of my pregnancy?
• Is there anything particular that you recommend that I do between now and the next time that I see you that is related to my stage of pregnancy?
• Do you recommend any complementary services or therapies? OR I have heard that ___ is particularly helpful. Would you recommend it and why?

Unless there is an emergency, it is always appropriate to ask questions and to ask to be given time to talk privately with your partner as you make a decision. Don't be afraid to come back in after a private chat and ask even more questions before making your final decision. Use the BRAT pack (described below) alongside this information so that you can ask the right questions at the right time. This questioning technique will also come in handy during labour, so practice it a lot during pregnancy. Be mindful of how you phrase your questions. Open questions usually elicit longer and more detailed answers, which are what you are looking for. Think about using phrases like, "How long?", "Tell me more?", "Can you describe?" and, "What do you mean?"

Closed questions usually elicit either a yes or no answer which does not necessarily explain the relevance or give you any more information.

Let's assume that your blood pressure is being checked.

You: "Is my BP normal?"

Nurse: "Yes."

This is a closed question - the answer could only be yes or no, and although you are relieved that your BP is normal, you really want more information to fully understand the relevance of checking your BP. A yes or no answer is usually not satisfactory when you want more details.

Ask an open-ended question like, "What information do you get from this reading and what is the relevance to my pregnancy?" or, "What does this reading mean?"

THE BRAT METHOD

There will also be times when an intervention is suggested. With every action, intervention, statement or procedure that you are not sure of, it is up to you to ask the right questions to get more information. For the purpose of this exercise, I am going to use induction of labour, but you can use this as an example for any situation where you feel uncomfortable or pressured to make a decision.

Let's say you get to 39 weeks and your doctor suggests doing an induction of labour. Admittedly you are fed up with being pregnant, feeling heavy and uncomfortable and totally ready. Your mother also arrives tomorrow and she is only staying for two weeks, so this could be really tempting. However, you have heard that having an induction sometimes leads to having a C-section and you would really prefer to have a natural birth. What you need is more information on the Benefits, Risks, Alternatives and Timing (BRAT). So ask questions like these:

What would be the BENEFIT, if any, of inducing my labour (or whatever your situation is)?
- benefit for me
- benefit for my baby
- benefit for you (the doctor)

Are there any RISKS associated with inducing labour (or whatever your situation is) at this stage of labour?
- risks for me
- risks for my baby
- risks for you (If you do/don't induce labour now)

Are there any ALTERNATIVES to doing a medical induction (or whatever your situation is) of labour?
- Are there any natural methods we could try?
- What is the success rate of these and how do they work?
- What are we trying to achieve and why?

What is the TIMING of this decision?
- How urgent is the situation?
- Will my health or the health of my baby be affected in any way by waiting?
- If not, how long could we safely wait and when will we reassess my situation?
- What criteria will you base your decision on?
- Is this an emergency?

These questions can be applied to any situation that you are faced with during your pregnancy and birth.

Questions to ask when a test or procedure is recommended:

- Is this test or treatment routine in pregnancy? How does it work?
- Why do I need it?
- What are the benefits to me or my baby?
- Are there any risks to me or my baby?
- Do I have to have it? If yes, do I need to do it now or can it be done later? Is timing important?

Questions to ask when medication is prescribed for any reason:

- What is the name of the medication you are prescribing?
- What is the reason you are prescribing it?
- Are there any potential risks or side effects that I should be aware of?
- What would happen if I chose not to take this medication?
- Are there any alternatives to this treatment?

A PDF summary of the BRAT method is available at www.thevirtualmidwife.com/resources.

UNDERSTANDING THE ROLE OF YOUR CARE PROVIDER

Learning the difference between various care providers that you will see throughout your pregnancy will guide you to know who to ask and to manage your expectations. Each person has a role in your pregnancy. Some of the roles cross over. Some roles can only be performed by the assigned care provider according to their skills and relevant expertise. You will see different people at different stages of your pregnancy.

During pregnancy:

• Take blood samples - the nurse at the clinic or the midwife.
• Do ultrasound scans - sonographer or your doctor.
• Check urine samples - the nurse at the clinic or the midwife.
• Check your blood pressure and weight - the nurse at the clinic or the midwife.
• Routine antenatal checkup - this will depend on the facility. It may be done by your midwife or by an obstetrician that you have chosen to see throughout your pregnancy. If you are at a public healthcare centre, it may be a different doctor every visit.
• Give antenatal information - the nurse at the clinic or the midwife. Some hospitals provide antenatal classes, however I highly recommend doing a private class that will include birth preparation skills and will be much more comprehensive and experiential. Most hospital classes are taught by the staff midwives and the information is limited to what to expect in the hospital rather than deep preparation for the challenges of birth.

During labour and birth:

• Provide medical assistance during labour - in public and private hospitals you will be attended throughout your labour by a staff midwife. In a birth centre, you will be attended by the midwife who followed your care throughout your pregnancy.
• Provide emotional support during labour - this will mainly be your partner and the staff midwife. I highly recommend hiring a doula who is trained to provide emotional support and nonmedical pain relief options to you throughout your labour. The presence of a doula at birth is proven to shorten labours and improve the maternal experience of labour and birth.
• Deliver the baby - this will be done by your midwife in a birth centre, by the staff midwife in a public hospital or by your obstetrician in a private hospital.
• Perform a C-section - a doctor.
• Know when a C-section might be required - all midwives are trained to know when to alert the doctor in the event of complications or things not progressing as expected.
• Perform episiotomy - all midwives are trained to do an episiotomy and to recognise when an episiotomy is required. They are also trained to suture them. Most episiotomies are done by doctors.
• Insert epidural - done by the attending anaesthetist (requires that you sign consent).
• Provide medical pain relief - midwives are trained to administer narcotics and to advise on the use of narcotic analgesia during labour. The most commonly used narcotic analgesia is pethidine and this needs to be prescribed by the doctor.

After birth:

Assist with breastfeeding - this is done by the staff nurses and midwives on the ward. If you are in a birth centre, the doulas are trained to assist you with breastfeeding. Some hospitals have staff lactation consultants. I highly recommend hiring a post-partum doula or lactation consultant to assist you during the first days with your newborn baby.

3. What to expect during pregnancy

Understanding the strange new sensations brought on by your pregnancy so you can be guided by them, rather than being afraid that something is wrong

COMMON DISCOMFORTS OF PREGNANCY

Many of the common discomforts of pregnancy would be an indication of something being wrong if you were NOT pregnant. However, in pregnancy they are normal and are occurring to prepare or protect you. This section will give you more insight into why they occur and how you can alleviate them by understanding them and working with them.

Pregnancy is a time of extreme self-care. The changes you will experience are an indication that your body is changing in response to your pregnancy. Now, more than ever, it is important for you to slow down and notice and respond to the changes. Remember that the changes and sensations that you experience are as a result of your pregnancy and have nothing to do with the fact that you are living abroad. It is the feelings that are foreign.

Breast changes

Oestrogen and progesterone are the chief pregnancy hormones that cause breast changes and you will produce more oestrogen during one pregnancy than throughout your entire life. Your body is gearing up for breastfeeding and the milk-producing glands are being stimulated.

Breast changes are usually the first signal that you may be pregnant and are usually noticeable around 4-6 weeks after conception. The slightest touch can be uncomfortable and sleeping face down is almost impossible. The discomfort usually eases as you enter the second trimester and may even disappear. During early pregnancy, small bumps known as Montgomery's tubercles will begin to appear on your areola. These are sebaceous glands that will secrete an oil to discourage bacteria and keep the areola and nipple protected and lubricated. These little bumps are often an early clue of a first pregnancy.

If your breasts go through a period of rapid growth, you may find that your breasts feel itchy as the skin stretches. Keeping the skin moisturised can help to relieve this discomfort. It is not uncommon for breast size to change in pregnancy. They may start to grow as early as week six and continue to the end of the pregnancy. The change could be slow, intermittent or rapid. Your ribcage will also expand towards the end of pregnancy, requiring a larger band size. Most women find that their bra size increases by at least a cup during their first pregnancy. You may develop stretch marks on your breasts, but these will usually fade over time. By the end of the pregnancy you will have up to 50 percent more blood in your body to meet the needs of your baby. The increased blood flow starts in early pregnancy to support your growing baby and can make the veins on your breasts more visible and prominent. The veins will become less noticeable after the birth, or when you stop breastfeeding. After this point, your breasts will not require an increased blood supply, and you should find the veins return to their pre-pregnancy state.

Backache

As your baby grows, the hollow in your lower back may become more pronounced, and this can also cause backache. During pregnancy, your ligaments become softer and stretch to prepare you for labour. This can put a strain on the joints of your lower back and pelvis, which can cause backache. Remember to bend your knees and keep your back straight when lifting or picking something up from the floor. Wear comfortable flat shoes during pregnancy to allow your weight to be evenly distributed. Always sit with your back straight and well supported.

Regular yoga practice keeps the muscles that support your back strong and flexible and eases daily aching. A firm mattress can help to prevent and relieve backache. If your mattress is too soft, put a piece of hardboard under it to make it firmer. Massage can help to increase the blood flow to the muscles. Very often backache can be caused by a pelvis that is out of alignment. Get this checked by a chiropractor. They will be able to give some advice and may suggest some helpful exercises.

Constipation

You may become constipated very early in pregnancy because of the hormonal changes taking place in your body. Eat foods that are high in fibre, like wholewheat breads, wholegrain cereals, fruits, vegetables and pulses such as beans and lentils. Drink plenty of water and exercise regularly to keep your muscles toned.

Cramp

Cramp is sudden, sharp pain, usually in your calf muscles or feet. It is most common at night. Nobody really knows what causes it, although it is thought to be related to a need for more calcium and potassium in the diet.

Regular, gentle exercise in pregnancy, particularly ankle and leg movements, will improve your circulation and may help to prevent cramps occurring.

Eat a banana daily and add almonds to your diet if you are experiencing cramp often and do daily yoga stretches to keep muscles strong and flexible while improving circulation.

Feeling faint

You may often feel faint when you are pregnant. This is because of hormonal changes taking place in your body. You are most likely to feel faint if you stand still for too long or get up too quickly from a chair or out of a hot bath. It can also happen when you are lying on your back. Try to get up slowly after sitting or lying down.

If you feel faint when standing still, find a seat quickly and the feeling should pass. If it doesn't, lie down on your side.

If you feel faint while lying on your back, turn on your side. It is advisable not to lie flat on your back at any time in later pregnancy or during labour.

Feeling hot

During pregnancy you are likely to feel warmer than normal. This is due to hormonal changes and to an increase in the blood supply to your skin. You are also likely to sweat more. Wear loose clothing made of natural fibres, as these are more absorbent and "breathe" more than synthetic fibres.

Headaches

Some pregnant women find they get a lot of headaches. Try to get more regular rest and relaxation.

Paracetamol in the recommended dose is generally considered safe for pregnant women but there are some painkillers that you should avoid. Speak to your pharmacist or doctor about how much paracetamol you can take and for how long.

Incontinence

Incontinence is a common problem. It can affect you during and after pregnancy.

Sometimes pregnant women are unable to prevent a sudden spurt of urine or a small leak when they cough, sneeze or laugh, or when moving suddenly or just getting up from a sitting position. This may be temporary because the pelvic floor muscles relax slightly to prepare for the baby's delivery.

Some women have more severe incontinence and find that they cannot help wetting themselves.

Indigestion and heartburn

Indigestion is particularly caused by hormonal changes and in later pregnancy by your growing uterus pressing on your stomach. Heartburn is more than just indigestion. It is a strong, burning pain in the chest caused by stomach acid passing from your stomach into the tube leading to your stomach. This is because the valve between your stomach and this tube relaxes during pregnancy. Sit up straight when you are eating, as this takes the pressure off your stomach.

Avoid the foods which affect you, for example, fried or highly spiced food, but make sure you are still eating well.

Heartburn is often brought on by lying flat. Sleep well propped up with plenty of pillows, and avoid eating and drinking for a few hours before you go to bed.

Your midwife may prescribe an antacid if the problem is persistent.

Itching

Mild itching is common to pregnancy because of the increased blood supply to the skin. In late pregnancy, the skin of the abdomen is stretched and this may also cause itchiness. Wearing loose clothing may help. Try natural clothing materials rather than synthetic materials.

Leaking nipples

Leaking nipples are normal and usually nothing to worry about. The leaking milk is colostrum, which is the first milk your breasts produce to feed your baby.

If your milk becomes bloodstained, see your doctor.

Nosebleeds

Nosebleeds are quite common in pregnancy because of hormonal changes. They don't usually last long but can be quite heavy. As long as you don't lose a lot of blood, there is nothing to worry about. You may also find that your nose gets more blocked up than usual.

Passing urine often

Needing to pass urine often may start in early pregnancy. Sometimes it continues right through pregnancy. In later pregnancy it is the result of the baby's head pressing on the bladder.

Pelvic joint pain

If during or after your pregnancy you have pain in your pelvic joints when walking, climbing stairs or turning in bed, you could have pelvic girdle pain (PGP) or symphysis pubic dysfunction (SPD). This is a slight misalignment or stiffness of your pelvic joints, at either the back or front. It affects up to one in four pregnant women to a lesser or greater extent. Some women have minor discomfort; others may have much greater immobility.

Getting diagnosed as early as possible can help to minimise the pain and avoid long-term discomfort. Treatment usually involves gently pressing on or moving the affected joints so they work normally again. Ask your doctor for a referral to a physiotherapist who is experienced in treating pelvic joint problems. These conditions tend not to get better completely without treatment from an experienced practitioner.

Piles

Piles, also known as haemorrhoids, are swollen veins around your anus (back passage) which may itch, ache or feel sore. You can usually feel the lumpiness of the piles around your anus. Piles may also bleed a little and they can make going to the toilet uncomfortable or even painful. They occur in pregnancy because certain hormones make your veins relax. Piles usually resolve within a week after birth. Eat plenty of food that is high in fibre, like wholewheat bread, fruit and vegetables. Drink plenty of water. This will prevent constipation, which can make piles worse.

Avoid standing for long periods and take regular exercise to improve your circulation.

Skin and hair changes

Hormonal changes taking place during pregnancy will make your nipples and the area around them go dark. Your skin colour may also darken a little, either in patches or all over. Birthmarks, moles and freckles may also darken. Some women develop a dark line from their belly buttons down to the top of their pubic hair. These changes will gradually fade after the baby has been born, although your nipples may remain a little darker.

If you sunbathe while you are pregnant, you may find that you tan more easily. Protect your skin with a good, high factor sunscreen. Don't stay in the sun for very long. Hair growth is also likely to increase in pregnancy. Your hair may also be greasier. After the baby is born, it may seem as if you are losing a lot of hair. In fact, you are simply losing the extra hair that you grew during pregnancy.

Sleep

Late in pregnancy it can be very difficult to get a good night's sleep. It can be uncomfortable lying down or, just when you get comfortable, you find that you have to get up to go to the toilet.

Some women have strange dreams or nightmares about the baby and about the birth. Talking about them can help. It might be more comfortable to lie on one side with a pillow under your tummy and another between your knees.

Stretch marks

These are pale lines which usually occur on your abdomen or sometimes on your upper thighs or breasts. Some women get them, some don't. It depends on your skin type. Some people's skin is more elastic. You are more likely to get stretch marks if your weight gain is more than average. It is very doubtful whether oils or creams help to prevent stretch marks. After your baby is born, the marks should gradually fade and become less noticeable.

Swollen ankles, feet and fingers

Ankles, feet and fingers often swell a little in pregnancy because your body is holding more water than usual. Towards the end of the day, especially if the weather is hot or if you have been standing a lot, the extra water tends to gather in the lowest parts of your body. Avoid standing for long periods and wear comfortable shoes. Put your feet up as much as you can, especially in the evening.

Teeth and gums

Bleeding gums are caused by a build-up of plaque (bacteria) on your teeth. During pregnancy, hormonal changes in your body can cause plaque to make your gums more inflamed. They may become swollen and bleed more easily. When your baby is born your gums should return to normal.

Tiredness

In the early months of pregnancy, you may feel tired or even desperately exhausted. The only answer is to try to rest as much as possible. Make time to sit with your feet up during the day and accept any offers of help from colleagues and family.

Towards the end of pregnancy, you may feel tired because of the extra weight you are carrying. Make sure that you get plenty of rest.

Vaginal discharge

Almost all women have more vaginal discharge in pregnancy. It should be clear and white and should not smell unpleasant. If the discharge is coloured or smells strange, or if you feel itchy or sore, you may have a vaginal infection. The most common infection is thrush, which your doctor can treat easily. You can help to prevent thrush by wearing loose cotton underwear.

Tell your doctor if you experience any of these symptoms. Also tell them if vaginal discharge or colour increases a lot in later pregnancy.

Varicose veins

Varicose veins are veins that have become swollen. The veins in the legs are most commonly affected. You can also get varicose veins in the vulva (vaginal opening). They usually get better after delivery. If you have varicose veins, try to avoid standing for long period of time and avoid sitting with your legs crossed.

Do foot exercises and other antenatal exercises such as walking and swimming, which help your circulation

NATURE'S SAFETY NETS

Regardless of where you are in the world, your wonderful body naturally adjusts and creates safety nets to keep you and your baby from harm. Sometimes these safety nets cause a bit of discomfort, which can make you worry that something is inherently wrong. They can also be represented as a problem by your doctor and a reason for interventions. Understanding them will help you to avoid unnecessary anxiety and guide you to use effective questioning to avoid unnecessary interventions.

Your cervix during pregnancy

Your cervix is literally the neck of the uterus, connecting the uterus to the vagina. It is made of fibrous, muscular tissue that feels firm to the touch, almost like touching the end of your nose.

If this is your first pregnancy, then your cervix has never opened before and in fact, its principal role during pregnancy is to stay closed.

Typically, it will be three to five centimetres long and naturally angled towards your back in what we call a posterior position. This prevents undue early pressure on the cervix, which could cause premature labour. You need to know this because it is not uncommon in some parts of the world for the doctor to do a vaginal examination at your 38/39-week checkup and to inform you with a worried look that your cervix is "very posterior" and that it is unlikely you will go into labour.

The power of suggestion can easily lead you to believe that something is inherently wrong with you. There isn't. Your cervix is doing what it is meant to do, and it is only a matter of time before it will soften and move more to the front (anterior). Throughout your pregnancy, your cervix does a wonderful job of staying closed and literally keeping your baby inside. The posterior position is perfectly designed to keep it closed by avoiding early undue pressure. If something like this happens to you, make sure that you reference the section on effective questioning techniques and use the BRAT method to have an open discussion and literally negotiate for more time.

In order for your baby to be born, the cervix needs to change function and open to allow the baby through. This occurs naturally towards the end of pregnancy as it starts becoming softer (called ripening) and shorter (called effacing) and this, coupled with increased downward pressure of your baby moving into position, will guide it to angle itself more towards the front part of your body or anterior.

A natural way of helping the cervix to soften, ripen and naturally move into a more favourable position is to have lots of really good sex. Semen contains the hormone prostaglandin which plays a major role in the softening of the cervix, and orgasm causes a rhythmic almost spasmodic contraction of the uterus that may well get things started.

As with everything in labour (and life), we have to look at the big picture. Nothing happens in isolation and many factors work together towards the one big event that is birth. The softening, effacement and dilation of your cervix is a necessary part of the process, but hormones, position of the baby and stage of pregnancy are all contributing factors and they all happen in the last four weeks of pregnancy. Adopt the pace of nature, not the pace of the doctor or the hospital.

Your cervix during labour

Having stayed closed and positioned towards your back throughout pregnancy, your cervix now moves into action and is a key player in your birth.

Under the influence of hormones it changes function completely and starts to become soft and more anterior so that it can be pulled UP and OPEN while your strong uterine muscles nudge your baby DOWN and OUT through the cervix and into your vagina. In traditional medical surroundings, we place a lot of emphasis on the dilation of the cervix and use it as a tool to gauge how your labour is progressing. Unfortunately, this puts a lot of pressure on you because many of the decisions will be made by time constraints dictated by norms of cervical dilation.

Most hospitals work with what we call a "partogram". Your labour progress will be charted on this graph and it is expected that your cervix will dilate at a rate of approximately 1 cm per hour after you reach 4 cm. This is completely unreasonable and unnatural. Having worked in labour rooms and used the partogram for years, I know that although this means that we expect you to be fully dilated within six to eight hours from four centimetres, you will ALL do it at your own pace. Some if you will putter along slowly and steadily. Some of you will stall periodically and then speed up. Some of you will just have hard, fast and incredibly intense labours. Some of you may require some medical assistance.

All of these would be normal. The cervix is just one of many factors that need to be considered. The other things that are just as important would be the rhythm and intensity of your uterine contractions/waves. How you are coping physically, emotionally and mentally. How relaxed or tense you are. What position you are comfortable in and the position of your baby as it descends and rotates through your pelvis.

During early labour, while you are still at home waiting for things to get going, you will not know how much your cervix is dilated and, to be honest, it does not matter. For as long as you are *in labour* (which means that you are experiencing rhythmic waves of sensation that become increasingly more intense as the intervals become shorter) your cervix will be changing constantly. With every uterine contraction, your cervix is changing on some level, whether it is just softening it or whether it is pulling it up a millimetre or centimetre. It is the job of the cervix to soften and open during labour, but it cannot happen in isolation.

During labour, your cervix and uterus work together as a team. If your uterus is not contracting, then your cervix is not opening. Putting too much emphasis on the number can affect your emotional state and your endurance. It can be so disheartening to hear that you are "only two centimetres" if you have been in early labour for days. Or on the flip side, you may be told you are eight centimetres, think that you are "almost there" and then experience a stall in your labour that makes you feel despondent.

Studies also show that vaginal exams are not always accurate. When you add in multiple people checking, the accuracy gets even worse. After all, it is an estimation based on experience and in many ways the size of the hand of the person who is checking. Often, I would have a doctor coming in to do a check soon after I had done one and give a completely different assessment. For instance, I would say six centimetres and they would say five. My patient would look at me with dismay and wonder how she went backwards? I could not tell you who was correct because it was an assessment, an estimation. The most important thing is to know if there is progress. Has there been a change since the last check? And, of course, the best person to assess change would be the person who did the last check.

I urge you to let go of the numbers and focus on what is happening in your body. When you are able to do this you will instinctively know what is happening and if the question is where to be, as in home or hospital, you will know when to leave home to go to the hospital and it will have nothing to do with knowing how many centimetres dilated you are. There are also other ways that will give you a much more accurate assessment.

The purple line

There is a natural line that starts at the anus and moves up the cleft between your buttocks. There is already a very faint line there during pregnancy, but it will be much more visible when you are in labour. In fact it will extend up as far as you are dilated. In other words, if it extends from the anus all the way up the cleft to the top of your buttocks, you can accurately assess that your cervix is fully dilated. If this is the case, it is highly probable that you will also be feeling a lot of pressure, as if you want to go to the toilet, and you will either be very vocal and "pushy" or very quiet and internally focused. Either way, you are deeply aware that your baby is ready to be born soon. Surprisingly this is a very effective way of assessing how far dilated you are without doing an internal vaginal examination.

According to a study done in 2010, published by BMC Pregnancy and Childbirth, the line seems to first show for most women around three to four centimetres. The further dilated a woman is, the more likely she is to have the line show up. The line shows up most when women are around seven to eight centimetres dilated, and seems to fade in some women at almost complete dilation, but is present at some point in labour for 76% of women. Now I am not suggesting that you are continuously checking your butt in the mirror during labour, but this would be a useful tool to use if you were unsure or if you wanted some reassurance when making a decision about moving to the hospital.

The purple line is believed to be due to the increased pressure on the veins around the sacrum which creates the dark line where the thin skin of the cleft can show it. This pressure from the head creating the line also means that you can reasonably assess the station of the baby's head as it moves down. Lower head = more pressure = higher line.

Your mucus plug

The mucus plug is the blobby sticky stuff that provides a natural barrier to infection at the mouth of the cervix. It is formed at the end of the first month of pregnancy when the ovum was implanted in your uterine cavity. The secretion of the cervical cells takes place on a continuous basis, ensuring that the plug is constantly replenished to fill the uterine cervix with no gaps between the uterine walls. The mucus contains antibodies which help the immune system to counteract pathogens.

It is roughly four to five centimetres long (when in the uterine cervix) or about two tablespoons (when it comes out) but, for most of you, it will come out in parts rather than as one single blob. You will notice that your discharge becomes particularly thick and sticky in the last weeks of pregnancy.

Although the colour is usually white-yellowish, it is often streaked with pink or brown and you may see streaks of blood. All these colours are considered variants of the norm, but as always, look at the big picture. If you had sex recently the discharge may contain remnants of semen. If you had a vaginal exam recently the discharge may contain streaks of blood. If you have been feeling stronger than normal contractions and you are near your due date, the expansion of the cervix can cause bursting of capillaries and spotting with the discharge. All of these would be considered normal and no cause for concern, but stay aware and observant.

The mucus plug (sometimes called "a show") passes in different ways and at different times. You may not even notice passing the mucus plug, especially if it plops out while you are on the loo. Sometimes it slides out when you are in the shower. Otherwise, you may see streaks of it in your underwear. The mucus plug will usually come away any time from 36 weeks onwards, in preparation for labour.

Most often it will come out three to five days before labour but can start coming away as early as two weeks before. If you see signs of the mucus plug, it is a sign that your cervix is softening, ripening, effacing, dilating and moving into position to give birth. It is an excellent sign. It does not mean you are in labour or even going into labour unless it is accompanied by contractions that are increasing in intensity and duration. It is normal to have increased vaginal discharge during pregnancy and usually it will be sticky, white or clear and odourless. If there is a strong smell and yellow or green discolouration, then seek a medical opinion to check if you have an infection.

Your uterus

Your uterus is probably the most incredible muscle in the body. Before pregnancy it is roughly the size of a small pear. By the time you have reached full term it has grown to accommodate a 3+ kg baby as well as a placenta and amniotic fluid. It then changes function completely to help you get the baby out!

A few years ago, I had a veterinary surgeon in one of my childbirth classes who was almost as passionate as me when it came to talking about the uterus. He summed it up perfectly by saying that it's the only organ in your body that can transform from a one-bedroom apartment into a hotel in nine months and soon after, transform back into a one-bedroom apartment! This is because your uterus has five very unique and amazing properties that influence labour and the muscle's effectiveness during birth – tone, contractility, retraction, fundal dominance, and rhythm.

1. Tone
Unlike other muscles like biceps and triceps that we can strengthen and tone by lifting weights or exercising, the muscles of the uterus are smooth muscle that you cannot consciously contract or tone. Research suggests that drinking red raspberry leaf tea during the last weeks of pregnancy helps to increase the tone of the uterus. This delicious tea is naturally high in magnesium, potassium, iron and B-vitamins, which makes it helpful for nausea, leg cramps, and improving sleep during pregnancy. The specific combination of nutrients in raspberry leaf make it extremely beneficial for the entire reproductive system. It strengthens the uterus and pelvic muscles and supports healthy blood vessel dilation, which helps during labour.

Studies have shown that women who take red raspberry leaf have a reduced incidence of birth interventions. Research has also found that women who drink red raspberry leaf tea regularly towards the end of their pregnancies have shorter second stages of labour than those who don't.

I suggest waiting until you are 34 weeks pregnant and then start by drinking one cup a day, and gradually increase this up to three or even four cups by the time you are 38+ weeks.

You can continue to drink the tea for two weeks after your baby is born to help your uterus shrink back down, boost your immune system, assist with milk supply and fight infection.

The taste of raspberry leaf is a little bitter, so you may want to sweeten it with some honey. If you're not a fan of fruit teas, you can also take red raspberry leaf in tablet form.

2. Contractility
Your uterus is made up of strong muscles. The middle layer, called the myometrium, is made up of three layers of smooth involuntary muscle. Muscles that are under your conscious control are called voluntary muscles, while muscles that are not under your conscious control are called involuntary muscles. In other words, you cannot control your contractions, just like you don't control the beating of your heart. This is very important to remember during labour. It is easy to be overwhelmed by the involuntary sensations of labour. It can make you feel out of control. If you accept that your body is doing what it is naturally designed to do and allow it to happen, you are able to work *with* it, rather than *against* it. When your baby is ready to be born, your uterus will begin contractions in response to chemical messages from the hormone oxytocin. This signals that your baby is getting ready to be born.

The muscles need to work really hard to pull the softened cervix up and over your baby's head. Think of pulling a turtleneck sweater over your head – the body of the sweater represents your uterus and the turtle neck is the cervix that opens and expands as your baby's head pushes through. The muscles work in two very distinct ways. The upper part, known as the fundus, is the most active part. The lower part is known as the passive segment. Your baby's head is in the lower part and its head is pressing down on your cervix. The longitudinal muscle fibres contract and gradually pull up the lower segment and cervix. They also gently nudge down on the baby, pushing it ever further into your pelvis and causing equal pressure on your cervix to help it dilate or open. So there is a dual action of pulling up and gently nudging down.

3. Retraction

If your uterus did not have this special ability, then your contractions would be useless. When you are in labour, the function of the uterine muscles is to draw up and open the cervix with rhythmic contractions of the longitudinal muscles. In order for the muscles to be able to maintain the increased dilation of your cervix, they also need to retract, rather than relax and let go. This means that the uterus can hold open the cervix, maintaining the increasing dilation. With each contraction, the cervix opens a little more. Between contractions, it maintains this opening through retraction and achieves further opening with the next contraction.

4. Fundal dominance

This might sound a bit scientific, but it refers to the spontaneous wave of movement moving downward through the uterus to help nudge your baby down and out. This fundal pressure increases at the end of labour when your baby is ready to be born, moving in a wave-like motion down the fibres of the uterus to encourage your baby's movement down and out. This is what I mean when I say that there is a dual action of pulling up (retraction) and nudging down (fundal dominance).

5. Rythm

Surprisingly, rhythm and harmony are essential for a smooth labour. Tension in the surrounding muscles causes resistance and disrupts the harmony of the muscle layers, causing irregular, sporadic contractions, rather than regular, rhythmic contractions. This results in what we call the fear/tension/pain cycle. Inherent fear causes you to tense up your muscles which in turn disrupts the harmony and rhythm of the involuntary muscles and results in true pain. This is why relaxation and breathing are so vital. Just like your mind and your body, each of the three layers of uterine muscle need to work together for efficient and comfortable movement.

Your amniotic fluid

This wonderful substance changes as your pregnancy progresses. It is initially created from your plasma and is mostly made up of water with electrolytes for the first 12 weeks. After this, proteins, carbohydrates, lipids and urea are present, providing essential nutrients for your baby to grow and develop as the fluid is absorbed into your baby's skin and tissue.

At around 16 weeks, your baby's kidneys begin to function and the skin begins to change. Your baby starts to "drink" the amniotic fluid rather than absorbing it and the kidneys process and excrete it back into the amniotic sac. Swallowing the amniotic fluid is an important developmental skill that your baby will start practising in utero in preparation for breastfeeding. The more they swallow, the more they pee, and by the end of the pregnancy, urine is the main source of amniotic fluid along with fluid excreted from your baby's lungs. Of course, amniotic fluid has some extremely important functions in pregnancy:
• cushions and protects your baby
• keeps a steady temperature around your baby
• helps your baby's lungs grow and develop because your baby breathes in the fluid
• helps your baby's digestive system develop because your baby swallows the fluid
• helps your baby's muscles and bones develop because your baby can move around in the fluid
• keeps the umbilical cord from being squeezed.

Vernix casseosa

This thick, white creamy substance coats your baby's skin during pregnancy and prevents him or her from pruning up in there. I mean, imagine soaking in a bathtub for nine months! It helps protect the delicate skin from the acidic quality of the amniotic fluid and helps keep infection at bay. It also has some other amazing properties that you need to know about:
• It is a lubricant that helps your baby slide down the birth canal a bit easier.
• It keeps your baby warm and helps to maintain a comfortable temperature in your belly.
• Only humans have it! No animals have vernix.
• It muffles sound, so although your baby can hear your voice by about 25 weeks, the vernix protects from loud noises.

• If your baby is overdue, the vernix will be scanty as most of it will have been absorbed into the amniotic fluid, but otherwise, you will see a thick coating after birth.
• It provides a protection to the skin. The WHO recommends delaying the first bath for 24 hours to allow the vernix to be absorbed into the skin.

Wharton's jelly

There are two arteries and a vein that transport blood between you and your baby via the placenta. This is the main connection keeping your baby alive and nurturing growth, so it's really important that it is well protected. This is the main role of Wharton's jelly, a clear, mucous tissue that insulates and protects the umbilical arteries and vein in the umbilical cord. It consists of mucopolysaccharides (fats), white blood cells, and stem cells. After birth, when the cord is exposed to the cooler temperatures outside your body, Wharton's jelly will collapse the venous structures within the cord and essentially cause a natural clamping, which occurs 5-20 minutes after birth. Cord clamping is not actually necessary at all, even though we do it. Despite what you see in the movies about having string and scissors available to tie off the cord, this is absolutely not necessary because of Wharton's jelly.

Rebecca's story

Rebecca called me at 11 a.m. to let me know that she was in early labour. Her first baby was a water birth in the UK and while she was not planning a water birth this time, we were both expecting a smooth and easy labour. When I got to her house, she was baking muffins and preparing to take her first daughter to a play date. We chatted for a while and then she took her daughter upstairs for a nap, and I encouraged her to stay with her and get some rest herself. An hour later, they both came downstairs all packed and ready to go to their play date.

I was a bit surprised that things seemed to have slowed down rather than picked up, and she was totally relaxed. Her husband arrived home from work and we decided that I would go and rest myself and she would call me when things picked up again.

Instinctively I felt that once things started, it would go quickly, so I ran some errands at a mall nearby. Barely an hour later, Clinton called me from his car and I could hear the unmistakable sounds of Rebecca pushing in the background. I told him to pull over and attend to her and raced to where they were. I got there in time for her baby boy to slide out gently into my hands in the back of their Porsche Cayenne parked outside the Royal Opera House in Muscat, Oman.

As soon as he was born, she started breastfeeding, and we set off for the hospital in heavy afternoon traffic. I left nature to do the rest, knowing that her breastfeeding would cause powerful contractions to stop the bleeding and separate the placenta. The cord naturally clamped as it cooled down, due to the nature of Wharton's jelly. Mom and baby were in absolute bliss.

4. Optimising health and wellness

Taking care of nutrition and other health issues for you and your baby

It goes without saying that a healthy diet is essential to grow a healthy baby. Your nutritional needs will change slightly during each trimester according to what your baby needs, but the most important thing to remember is to maintain a daily diet that includes tasty, nutrient-rich foods.

You may find that your tastebuds change a lot during pregnancy. It is not unusual to find yourself wanting to eat foods that you previously disliked or not being able to stomach foods that you usually love.

I have worked with several happy vegetarians who suddenly found themselves craving meat during pregnancy. My favourite was Lindsey, who had been a vegetarian for well over a decade when she got pregnant. Her craving to eat meat was so bad that she made herself watch reruns of the movie that originally inspired her to become vegetarian. But it did nothing. All she could think of was meat and she eventually gave in and ordered her husband to the store to buy her some steak. She ate meat three times a week for the rest of her pregnancy and it just felt right. Six months after her daughter was born, she went back to being a happy vegetarian, but the same thing happened when she got pregnant again with her son, and this time she went with it.

I truly believe that your body will tell you what you need and how much. Eat well. Make healthy choices. Listen to your body. By following some fairly easy nutrition guidelines, you will have a healthy pregnancy. I will not go into too much detail about diet in this book as it would be another book altogether and there have been recent advances that you need to be aware of. Conventional prenatal nutrition advice can be misleading and it is important that you follow a nutrient-dense diet that includes key nutrients for your baby's development. Many of these are found in the very foods you're told to limit by conventional prenatal nutrition guidelines. I have some book recommendations on my website that I highly recommend in order to get the latest research-based evidence regarding a healthy pregnancy lifestyle plan, but I will outline some of the essentials here.

THREE ESSENTIAL NUTRIENTS AND WHY THEY ARE IMPORTANT

Iron

Iron is important to maintain a healthy haemoglobin (Hb) level. We expect a level of between 10-14 g per decilitre (dL) to maintain a healthy pregnancy, so it is important to include iron-rich foods in your diet and to take a prenatal supplement that contains adequate iron.

Iron-rich foods include brussel sprouts, sunflower seeds, apricots and tomatoes.

Folate

Folate is a general term for a group of water-soluble B-vitamins. It is also known as B9. Folic acid refers to the oxidized synthetic compound used in dietary supplements and food fortifications. There is a difference between the naturally occurring folate and the synthesised folic acid. I highly recommend staying as natural as possible by including folate-rich foods in your diet and taking a prenatal supplement that provides two critically important forms of folate: folinic acid and methylfolate.

Folate-rich foods include asparagus, parsley, cauliflower and beets. Iron and folate-rich foods include spinach, collard greens, broccoli and turnip greens.

Calcium

Calcium builds strong bones and encourages proper function of the muscular and nervous systems. It is also important to support the circulatory system so that nutrients are efficiently delivered to your baby.

Calcium-rich foods include dairy products, salmon, sesame seeds, kale, dried figs, molasses, oranges and almonds.

WHAT ABOUT MORNING SICKNESS?

Whether you are in your home country or abroad, morning sickness is a normal part of pregnancy and almost 50% of women experience some form of nausea and extreme fatigue during the first trimester. Although it usually peaks in the morning and eases as the day goes on, it can occur at any time of the day, and for some unfortunate women it continues throughout the day. I truly believe that it is a strong signal from your body to slow down. The reason you feel so rotten is that all your systems are in overdrive as everything kicks in to nurture your new pregnancy. Take heed and take rest.

For most women it may stop around the 12th week of pregnancy. The challenge is to get sufficient nutrition when eating is the last thing in the world that you feel like doing. The biggest concern is the effect it may have on your growing baby. Remember that your body compensates for this by drawing nutrients and energy from your stores - so this is why you will feel even more awful and absolutely exhausted. Remember that it will pass and, of course, if it is really bad, you will need to be admitted to get intravenous hydration. There is also a range of prenatal vitamins in spray form that are immediately absorbed sublingually if you are concerned that you are constantly vomiting your prenatal vitamins up and not getting the full benefit.

Helpful tips for morning sickness

- Snack frequently and nap when you feel tired.
- Drink fluids half an hour before or after a meal, but not with meals.
- Eat soda crackers 15 minutes before getting up in the morning.
- Eat whatever you feel like eating, whenever you feel you can, even if it is just a few mouthfuls.
- Avoid warm places (feeling hot adds to nausea).

Top 10 snacks when morning sickness strikes

You may find that there is just one thing that you can tolerate during this time and it is quite likely that it has little or even no nutritional value. While this is not ideal, go with it, but try and include the following 10 foods that are simple and easy to digest.

1. **Applesauce:** Cook up a few peeled apples and mash them up with some cinnamon and a sprinkle of nutmeg. Freeze in ice cube trays so that you have small tasty bites that you can either suck on or defrost and eat a few spoons to settle your tummy.

2. **Bananas:** These are rich in potassium, folate and vitamin B6 and I recommend including a banana a day throughout your pregnancy if you can. They are great on their own and very versatile in smoothies and deserts.

3. **Broth:** This is an excellent supplement throughout your pregnancy and particularly in the 4th trimester when you are establishing breastfeeding. Commit to making a large pot and freezing small quantities that you can drink like a cup of tea or stir an egg through to add to the nutritional value. It is an excellent source of sodium and potassium if you use lots of bones and vegetables to add variety and increase the overall nutritional value.

4. **Brown rice:** Sometimes you want something really bland and brown rice ticks all the boxes while still giving you B-vitamins and plenty of fibre. Add a teaspoon of coconut oil to bump up the nutritional value.

5. **Ginger:** Versatile and tasty, ginger is renowned for combating nausea and can be used in several ways. Grate it into boiling water to make a tea, add it to a smoothie or chew on a fresh piece of organic ginger.

6. **Ice chips:** Some women actually crave the crunch of ice. If this is you, then make ice out of ginger and lemon water or even frozen watermelon or cucumber juice. They are all bland but may give you the hit you need and combat the nausea.

7. **Lemons:** Along with ginger, lemons are great at combating nausea and they are rich in vitamin C. Nibble on slices, suck on segments, add them to your tea or pile them up in cool water with some fresh mint.

8. **Oatmeal:** If you are feeling brave and need something warm and hearty, then oatmeal offers protein, vitamins and minerals and can settle a funny tummy. Great with a swirl of honey and some sliced banana and some chopped dates or strawberries.

9. **Popcorn:** Not just for movies, popcorn is a whole grain with a good amount of fibre and is easy to nibble on throughout the day. Sprinkle generously with salt if you need to replace sodium from vomiting.

10. **Watermelon:** If this is in season and available when morning sickness strikes, you are in luck. It is packed with B-vitamins, lycopene, vitamin C, vitamin A and fibre. It is also rich in antioxidants which help with your energy levels! Freeze chunks to suck on or make a watermelon slushy to sip on slowly.

HEALTHY WEIGHT GAIN DURING PREGNANCY

Once you are over the morning sickness, focus on maintaining a healthy, balanced diet. There is so much emphasis on weight gain and looking perfect that sometimes we have unrealistic expectations. Remember that you are expected to gain weight and the rate and amount will have a lot to do with your starting weight and your general metabolism. You may gain less if you are overweight to start with, or more if you are underweight to start with, but you SHOULD gain weight.

As a general rule:
• If you are underweight with a body mass index (BMI) of less than 19 you should gain 12.5-18 kg (28-40 lb).
• If you have a BMI of 20-26 you should gain between 12-16 kg (25-35 lb).
• If you are overweight with a BMI of 27-30 you should gain between 7-11 kg (15-25 lb).
• If you have a BMI above 30 you should gain 7 kg or less (15 lb).

The weight gain is attributed to the changes in your breasts (8%), placenta (9%), uterus (11%), amniotic fluid (11%), increased blood volume (22%) and your baby (39%).

EXERCISE DURING PREGNANCY

Like weight-gain during pregnancy, knowing what kind of exercise and how often to do it will depend on your fitness level when you became pregnant. Pregnancy is not the time to embark on a rigorous fitness programme. This is not to say you have permission to be a couch potato, but rather that you should listen to your body and do exercises that feel good, suit your body type and are suitable for pregnancy.

I have worked with women across the entire spectrum of being super fit athletes to finding a daily walk difficult. The super fit are accustomed to a daily regime and their mindset is to push their body to the limits and beyond. While this is a great mindset to have in labour, I sometimes have to gently guide them to ease back and shift gears to focus on their changing body and to be more mindful of what is happening within. With these women, the focus is on physical exertion and fitness. During pregnancy you need to turn within and be mindful of your growing baby. Think about becoming "birth fit" and working from the inside out, rather than the outside in.

On the flipside, I have noticed that the women who have no former exercise routine revel in getting to know their bodies and feeling the changes that are happening as they get birth fit.

My personal exploration into yoga was fuelled after seeing the benefits while working in the labour room. I noticed that the women who had an established prenatal practice had shorter labours, managed the sensations better and used breathing techniques to full effect. I would gauge that 70% of the women who attend my prenatal yoga classes have never done any form of yoga before and most of them are hesitant to join but do so because it is known to be safe and effective. I love watching their confidence grow and hearing feedback (very often from their husbands) of how much better it makes them feel overall.

One of the many reasons that yoga is so beneficial is that your body is flooded with the hormone relaxin during pregnancy. This hormone is responsible for so many of the discomforts and challenges and, as the name suggests, it is responsible for relaxing all your systems. I encourage you to do the same and relax-in to the effects of relaxin rather than resisting. You may notice that you are more flexible than before. This is a direct result of relaxin which softens the joints and ligaments of the pelvis allowing it to accommodate the passage of your baby's head during birth. Unfortunately, during pregnancy it can cause pain in the pelvic joints and hips. Yoga stretches and strengthens muscles, so a regular practice will help you to avoid or alleviate these symptoms with poses commonly referred to as hip openers.

Relaxin allows the abdominal muscles to soften and stretch as your belly expands but also inhibits uterine contractions during the early stages of the pregnancy, which prevents premature labour. The breathing exercises and techniques that you learn in prenatal yoga will help you to strengthen your abdominal muscles and you will learn to use them effectively during pushing.

Relaxin affects the rib cage so that the body can better adjust to the pressure on the diaphragm from your growing uterus, but this is why you feel breathless, especially in the second trimester. Once again, the breathing techniques will make your more aware of your diaphragm and will teach you how to breathe effectively to minimise the discomfort of your growing belly.

Relaxin makes your bowel movements slow and sluggish, which can lead to constipation.

Obviously, this impacts the way you digest food and how you feel after eating. Yoga poses aid digestion and keep things moving along. I also recommend daily walking or a gentle swim to get your circulation going and stimulate digestion.

You might notice an increase in saliva as your pregnancy progresses. This helps the food break down more quickly before it reaches the colon. Your stomach capacity will shrink as it is pushed out of the way, so you will find that you will need to eat smaller meals more frequently to stay well nourished and avoid feeling full and uncomfortable.

Tips for constipation caused by relaxin:

• A tablespoon of organic cold-pressed coconut oil added to every meal or used during cooking is not just an excellent source of healthy fats but will soften and lubricate your stools.

• Treat constipation with a tablespoon of psyllium husk added to a glass of warm water before bed. Psyllium husks are a natural fibre which will move through your digestive tract and soften your stool.

• Stewed dried fruit (especially prunes and apricots), with a dollop of probiotic yoghurt, is another excellent and tasty way of treating mild constipation.

• Make sure you are drinking enough water to keep your stools well hydrated and keep your digestive tract active.

• Warm water with lemon is particularly effective.

SUPPLEMENTS

Despite a healthy diet and exercise program, you will need prenatal supplements to ensure that you are getting the recommended daily allowance (RDA) of essential vitamins and minerals. There are many brands available, and it can be hard to know which to choose. I recommend any brand that includes a range for each trimester as your needs will change as your pregnancy progresses. If you are suffering from extreme vomiting, you may consider a spray form of prenatal vitamins that is absorbed under the tongue.

5. Mental and emotional preparation

The internal work of preparing to become parents

Consider how you might have felt had you found out you were pregnant while still back in your home country, surrounded by family and loved ones. While you would still have experienced the same fears about giving birth, they would be dampened by the perceived safety of a known environment and the proximity of loved ones. Being pregnant for the first time, in a foreign healthcare system, far from support, can easily alter your experience from one of excitement to one of anxiety. Fear can very easily get in the way of a positive birth.

This chapter is about learning to let go of factors out of your control and focusing on those that are. Fear is fundamental to life on earth and is necessary to protect us against perceived or real threat. The same chemicals that contribute to the "fight or flight" response can also evoke feelings of happiness and excitement. Both of them are states of high arousal, but there is a difference between paralysing fear and a rush of happiness.

The way you experience fear has a lot to do with the context. Regardless of where you are, I urge you to treat your pregnancy as a life event, an adventure, an opportunity for deep transformation. Your pregnancy (the process of growing a baby in your body) will not be any different because of your geographical location. Your body will just get on and do what it knows how to do.

The perception of feeling in control is vital in understanding how you experience and respond to fear. When you recognise that being pregnant is a natural and normal state and rename and reframe your fears, you will be able to regain your sense of control and your confidence in your ability to confront the factors that initially scared you. If you want to enjoy your pregnancy and co-create a positive and memorable birth experience, you first have to address the world within. The external conditions you're confronted with - living in a strange land with different language, culture and customs - will seldom change, if you do not change the internal.

Your mind holds great potential to change and influence the way you live. The power of your mind is largely dependent on your thoughts. The old cliché that says you become what you think about holds true even in the context of pregnancy and birth.

Your beliefs, mindsets and attitudes influence how you behave and how you respond to certain events. Even more so, your thought patterns largely decide how you interpret certain situations. This can make the difference between seeing your situation as hopeless, horrible and frightening to embracing it as an adventure and an opportunity for growth as you transition to parenthood. Two people might share exactly the same experience, but the way they perceive, interpret and respond to their situation determines the outcome. This means you need to examine and reframe your fears, whether perceived or real.

Your brain is made of two distinct hemispheres, and while both hemispheres are skilled in all areas, each hemisphere is dominant in certain activities. The only barrier to expressing and applying all of these skills is your knowledge of how to access them.

The left hemisphere is the thinking, decision-making, logical side of the brain, and this is the part that is going to be particularly active during pregnancy. This is the part that is active right now while reading and analysing my words, storing new information and searching back to access prior learning and memories to put the information into context. The right hemisphere is the intuitive, emotional and creative side of your brain and it is the part of the brain that is most active during birth because birth is not about analysing and thinking. Giving birth is an act of BEING rather than DOING. This requires allowing the left, thinking side to almost shut down in order to allow the right, intuitive side to take over.

Pregnancy is the time to DO stuff. Labour and birth is the time to BE. It is a necessary process of letting go and allowing, naturally aided by hormones and the natural rhythms of labour. You will not be able to get into this right-sided intuitive and almost primal state if you fight to stay in control and keep doing. This will take some practice and forms a valuable and necessary part of your birth preparation.

LEFT-BRAIN PREPARATION (DOING)

Here are some of the left-brain activities you can do to prepare yourself:
- Researching pregnancy and birth-related topics online and in person.
- Educating yourself about what to expect.
- Learning about the stages of labour - what happens, how long does it take, how does it feel?

• Learning the signs that indicate when to go to the hospital, the signs of labour, and what it might feel like.
• Learning the physiology of labour: What are contractions and why are they necessary?
• Learning the anatomy of your body: Your cervix and how it dilates, the muscles of the uterus and how they work to dilate the cervix, the bones of the pelvis and how the baby fits through them.
• Learning about how the "pain" of labour is different from any other pain you may have experienced and the many ways you can prepare and cope with it.
• Researching and learning to understand the hospital system and how to deal with doctors, interventions and care practices.

RIGHT-BRAIN PREPARATION (BEING)

Here's how you can make use of the creative and instinctive side of your brain:
• Creating your "best birth for me" story - a free writing exercise to allow your subconscious to bring forth your beliefs and expectations.
• Keeping a journal of thoughts, reflections, fears, insights and revelations, in your own words, without judgment or the need to explain or defend.
• Allowing yourself to daydream without limits. Finding what works for you, what resonates, what feels right and good. Accessing trust.
• Using your left-brain acquired information to create and practise a visualisation of your birth.
• Learning to trust strange and uncomfortable sensations. Getting to know your body.
• Learning about your breath. Taking time every day to practise conscious breathing and exercising being present with uncomfortable sensations.
• Being able to get a mental picture of your baby in your belly and taking time daily to place your loving and undivided attention on this deep connection that is growing. Learning to listen, feel, connect and communicate with your baby in this unique way.
• Listening to your inner dialogue and learning to discern between learned thoughts, everyday chatter, and inner wisdom. What is your wisdom saying to you? How does it make you feel? Are you able to trust it? How will you learn to balance it with the external influences, facts and opinions?

FEAR IN PREGNANCY

There is a lot of fear surrounding birth in the 21st century. I would venture to say that fear is one of the most prevalent emotions I encounter in my work with women and birth. Fear is fuelled by stories you hear from friends and relatives sharing their not so perfect birth stories. It is compounded by doing internet searches on common discomforts of pregnancy and skipping through to the worst-case scenario.

A lot of the information you read will trick you into believing things that are not real or true. In fact, that is exactly what fear is - False Evidence Appearing Real. Fear begins in the mind. It is not something you can feel, touch or see. It is not a thing. It is so easy to always see the dark side of things, especially when you are in situations that are out of your comfort zone.

Instead of embracing pregnancy as a beautiful life event and milestone, you see it as a minefield of dangerous choices and decisions. Stopping this is not just about having a good attitude or being positive just for the sake of being positive, although this definitely has benefits. You will need to become more aware of what you think and recognise that how you think directly affects the things that happen to you. If you do not take the time and make the effort to discover and face your fears during pregnancy, they will surface during labour and impact the way that you experience the sensations of labour and your birth experience. Your mindset will determine whether you are able to approach labour as intense and challenging or hold onto your perception of it being painful and frightening. Which would you prefer?

Your mind is open, and you are the only one who is responsible for ensuring that it does not become a mass of insecurities fueled by neglect and negative thought patterns. Any imbalance caused by fear in the emotional right brain and the sense of control in the contextual left brain can cause too much or not enough excitement. If you perceive your situation as too real, too fearful, too extreme, you sense a loss of control over your situation.

Bear in mind that whenever we respond to an event there is an element of "how you feel" and "what you think". Where do these two intersect and which one are you going to place your focus on?

The way you feel usually relates to your intuition, gut feeling or body wisdom. What you think relates to what you see and hear and the way that your brain will search your memory bank, much like going through a filing cabinet, to find a similar situation or event to guide your response. If it cannot find the relevant information that it is looking for it will guide you to read and research more so that you can respond with confidence and competence.

As a modern, educated woman you are part of a generation that is used to being in control of your life and at work. You may find it difficult to let go and accept that birth is a process that cannot be managed like a work project. A large part of this process involves letting go of:
• Negative beliefs, for example: "I will never be able to give birth safely in this country."
• Limiting beliefs, for example: "I just know that my pain tolerance level is low and I won't be able to cope."
• Cultural conditioning, for example: "Giving birth is inherently dangerous."
• Factors out of your control, for example: environmental, obstetric or anatomical.

The reaction of fear begins in your brain and rapidly spreads throughout your body, preparing you to flee or defend yourself. It begins in a region of your brain called the amygdala which is dedicated to detecting the emotional importance of the stimuli.

Imagine that you are having your first scan. You are excited to see your baby for the first time and anxious about any other information you might get at the scan. You notice that the ultrasonographer is staring intently at the screen and not saying a word; her eyes are wide and she is not smiling. The sight of her face triggers a fear response and your mind immediately assumes the worst. Your amygdala detects an emotional response that triggers a physical response and release of stress hormones, assuming that she is about to deliver bad news. Your brain becomes hyperalert, your pupils dilate and your breathing accelerates. Your heart rate and blood pressure rise. All of this happens purely in response to a perceived threat. She has not said or done anything to make you fearful, it's only her bedside manner that is somewhat lacking. In your anxiety, you have perceived her behaviour as a prelude to bad news, all based on assumption. A moment later she smiles, turns the screen around and points out your perfect baby with everything normal and intact. Your fear was imagined, but your response was real. Your mind does not know the difference between imagination and reality. But you do.

You control your rational mind. You control your rate and depth of breathing. When you move into fear by allowing irrational thoughts, your body releases adrenaline and sends you into a state of panic, alerting you to fight, freeze or flee. Your mind controls your body. So ultimately, you control your fear and your ability to confront or move beyond your fear. You control how you experience your pregnancy, your interactions with people and the intensity of your birth experience.

I have identified 10 common fears based on my experience of working with women during pregnancy:
1. I will lose control.
2. I will be separated from my baby or partner.
3. I won't feel supported.
4. I won't be able to stand the pain.
5. I won't be able to relax.
6. My baby is too big or my pelvis is too small.
7. I won't have privacy.
8. My cervix won't dilate.
9. I'll have to fight to have my wishes respected.
10. I'll be given interventions that may not be necessary.

Do you have any other fears that are not included here? What are they? I encourage you to spend some time examining these statements and reframing them by asking yourself the following questions:
• Is this fear based on external factors out of my control?
• Is this fear based on an assumption? (do you know it to be true? Where did you hear this from?)
• Is this fear based on a limiting belief?
• Is this fear based on factual evidence?
• What can I do to reframe or eliminate this fear?

You will be surprised that many of them (if not all of them) are based on assumptions, limiting beliefs and factors out of your control. Doing this exercise will not necessarily eliminate your fears, but it will highlight them and help you to reframe them and manage them more effectively.

When I first started working independently in Oman I had two clients who approached me, both wanting a water birth. No water births had ever been done in Oman and there was no hospital that had the facilities or even the staff. It was really not an option and I told them both as much, but also said that perhaps it had never been done because nobody had asked, and that it was worth investigating further. I also told them both that I would do whatever I could to support them.

The one client, Molly, did a bit of research and asking about, but seemed to give up on the idea in the face of the unenthusiastic response she received. Lindsay, however, was determined and just kept asking, going back again and again and doing the research on how to make it happen. She spoke to all the doctors and hospitals and eventually went ahead and bought her own inflatable "pool in a box". The staff and doctors did everything they could to dissuade her, but her mind was set. Two months later, a new midwife with considerable experience in water birth started at the hospital she had chosen and the wheels started turning. She got her water birth and three years later she took it one step further and had a home birth, which was also unheard of at the time (and still is).

The two attitudes can be summed up in these statements:

"I wanted a water birth but they told me it wasn't possible."

"I wanted a water birth and they told me it wasn't possible, but I did my research, stood by my decision and made it happen."

Lindsay's story in her own words

I would like to share my experience of preparing for and giving birth in Oman. I began my prenatal care at one of the two private hospitals I had chosen, but in the end it couldn't give me what I wanted. I think the most important thing that women here need to remember is that you are in control of your birth experience. Ask questions. Do the research if you have any complications and don't be afraid to challenge your doctor and/or change doctors or hospitals in order to get what you want. I wanted a water birth and was told I couldn't have one, until the end of my pregnancy came around and it was time to really discuss the details. I didn't care for the midwife I met, my doctor was going on holiday around my due date and the backup doctor I wanted was so busy my chances of getting her were slim, so with all that stacked up against me I changed hospitals at 37 weeks. I bought my own pool, which I ordered from the UK and had brought over. We were the second water birth at that hospital.

I would also advise meeting the midwives employed by the hospital and to hire your own labour support. The hospital midwives are going to be with you for the bulk of your labour and bringing your own labour support ensures you won't ever be alone and also provides your husband with help should he need it. Make sure everyone knows what you want so you can trust your birthing team, trust your birthing space and therefore trust birth itself. I put a lot of work into mentally preparing for the big day. There are many different methods to choose from. I liked HypnoBirthing by Marie Mongan and faithfully practised relaxation techniques throughout my third trimester. Prenatal yoga also helped me practise slow, steady breath. I made a vision board, posted affirmations around my flat, allowed myself to feel scared, explored my options if I just couldn't do it and basically prepared for birth as I would an exam. I truly believe all this preparation manifested the birth that I wanted and thankfully nothing out of my control prevented that. I trusted birth and knew I could do it. There is a quote that stayed with me throughout my pregnancy and birth and that is, "The contractions cannot get bigger than you, because they are you."

I knew my baby was going to be born the night before its birth because at yoga class I couldn't get into any of the positions I normally could, and sure enough, the next morning things got started. I woke up feeling as though my period was about to start and there was a bloody show. I was one week overdue but not really sure if I was in labour. My water didn't break until I was in my birthing pool. I kept myself busy. I cleaned the house, baked a cake, prepared dinner and then took a nap. I woke up at 1 p.m. to more intense cramping coming in waves. I was very surprised that I didn't feel it in my baby bump at all. The sensations were down low in my pelvis. I discovered my mantra, "Down, baby down", as I bounced and rolled on the birth ball. My husband, Bobby, was so calm and cool. He timed my contractions and held onto me middle-school slow dance style while he rubbed my back. In between the cramps, I had to use the toilet a lot. I had an appointment scheduled that day at 4 p.m. but cancelled and let the hospital know I would probably be coming in later that evening. My midwife/doula, Karen, came around 5 p.m.

and sat with me while my husband put the dinner in the oven, walked the dog, loaded the car, etc. I tried to listen to the HypnoBirthing visualisations my husband had recorded for me, but at that moment they were a distraction. I did a good job on my own, staying with my breath and keeping my body relaxed. I was in the zone. Then I had a huge vomit and thought I was going to go take a nap. HA! I lay down for 30 seconds and was like, "Right, let's go."

I lay in the back seat of the car and repeated my plan to myself; I would walk upstairs to the maternity ward, sit on the toilet and get in my pool. Which is exactly what I did. Bobby and Karen set up my pool, while we waited for the hospital midwife on duty, Kaya, to examine me. I said in my birth plan that I didn't want to know how many centimetres I was because I didn't want to be disappointed, so I wasn't told but it turns out I was 9 centimetres when I got to the hospital! I got in the pool at 8 p.m. and it felt amazing. My team totally respected my wishes. It was dark and quiet with relaxing dream pop music in the background. There was no screaming or freaking out. At the end, I did feel some fear. I was surprised I felt it so much in my bum. It's pretty intense. At one point I told the room I was feeling a little lazy and needed a break. After a pep talk from Karen, I had a bit of a yell as I pushed her head out while I was on all fours in my water pool. My doc was surprised when I said it's out. Then Kaya told me to roll back and the rest of her came out and she was on my chest just like that. We didn't know if she was a boy or a girl for nearly a full minute. I asked Bobby, "Is it a boy or a girl?" and he said he didn't know and that they were waiting for me to tell. It was a girl (Zahrada Theodora). "It's a girl! Zazie is here!" What an amazing experience!

As soon as my daughter was out, all the pain went away. I was on a natural high. We got to cuddle her for a minute and had plenty of time to allow the cord to stop pulsing before it was cut. My husband went with another midwife, Sam, and our daughter to get her checked out, measured weighed etc. while I got out of the pool to deliver the placenta. I also got a small tear and needed stitches. It will be my goal for my next baby to stay relaxed even at the end, but then again she was 8 pounds 9 ounces (or 4.04 kilograms) so whatever. I left the hospital the next day feeling so good about my birth experience.

———

For every reason that you think it might not be possible, there are always people who have faced the same circumstances and succeeded. I am always amazed when people argue for their limitations. It is not the limiting factors that are limiting you - it is you.

It is up to you to change the way that you respond to the events and circumstances you are faced with to get the outcomes that you want. You may need to change your way of thinking, the words you use when you are communicating ideas, change your thoughts, your behaviour and the pictures you hold in your mind. But you have control over all of these things. You CAN change them.

You cannot change the hospital system, or the fact that you are living on a different continent to your family, or the language and culture of your host country - but you can change your response to these circumstances. You can learn about the hospital system so that you can work with it (rather than against it). You can use technology to stay in touch with your family and see it as an adventure and a challenge. You can learn more about the language and culture of your host country or at least make sure that you have a translator with you when you go for doctor's appointments and routine tests and scans.

The bottom line is that YOU are the one who is creating your life the way that it is. The country, job and situation that are living right now is the result of past thoughts, choices and actions. You are responsible for what you say, what you feel, what you do, what you choose to read and what you choose to believe. Having a baby is a life experience. Not a medical event. You are in charge of how it will unfold. And it all starts in the mind with your thoughts, beliefs and behaviour.

If you believe that a positive birth experience is possible, then make it happen. Shift your perspective on the external factors and examine your internal influences and resources. Everything you think, say, and do needs to become intentional and aligned with your purpose, your values and your goals. A positive birth experience is one where you confidently participate in all the choices and decisions during pregnancy and birth. The way your baby is born is important but either way, your baby WILL be born one of three ways:

1. You will go into labour (spontaneously or induced) and give birth vaginally.

2. You will go into labour (spontaneously or induced) and require an emergency C-section.

3. You will have an elective (planned) C-section.

Plan for the birth experience that you desire. Prepare for the birth experience that may occur due to factors that are out of your control. A positive birth experience is one that you will look back on with fond memories and be able to note the different twists and turns that occurred, many unexpectedly. You will be able to reflect on how you responded in a way that guides you to know what you would do the same next time, and what you might do differently. There will be some things you might wish you had known and others that you wish someone had told you. But, your overall memory is a positive one, your sense of satisfaction and achievement is high. Prepare yourself for a positive birth experience.

Lindsey and Tim Hounsom's birth story in their own words

We were from the UK and on a military three-year posting to Oman. I got pregnant in Muscat, Oman, and gave birth in Muscat too.

I knew, if things worked out for us, that we would be pregnant and giving birth in Oman during our military posting. I felt a bit daunted by the prospect of giving birth abroad, and had no idea how the system worked. I was lucky to live in a military compound, where other couples had already experienced the medical system. Most had been through the local military hospital for their care. On talking to them, I was more daunted and scared by the fact that the local system involved long waits, no consistency with medical staff, and mixed messages regarding results/scans that they'd had. For that reason, we chose to use the private system. It was within this system that you were guaranteed to see the same doctor throughout, have less of a wait for each appointment, and I'd heard good things about the medical staff. I felt more confident using this system, and we were fortunate to have the money to do so. I thought the whole pregnancy package was very reasonable regarding cost.

I developed high blood pressure during my pregnancy, so was on medication for the last part of my pregnancy. I had been taking my blood pressure myself, so I was the one that brought this up to the doctor. Otherwise, I'm not sure this would have been picked up as quickly. It might well have been picked up a bit quicker in the UK, with the more frequent appointments from the local midwife service.

During the pregnancy, we sourced private antenatal classes with Karen. I had known about the classes as I was attending Karen's pregnancy yoga classes (I still miss those!). I know in the UK we would have received these classes through the NHS or a similar private company. I'm not sure whether I'd have known about the classes had I not been attending the yoga. At the time, the private hospital didn't offer antenatal classes.

I was in a lovely local hotel when I went into labour. Six hours later Isaac was born at the private hospital. I was lucky my labour was quick and uncomplicated and I was fully dilated on reaching the hospital. He was three weeks early, so interrupted our lovely weekend away unexpectedly! The midwife staff were awesome and I have to say, since giving birth in the UK with my second child, the care I received in the hospital was far better than in the UK. The only thing I would say is that the staff wanted me on my back for the birth, which was really quite uncomfortable as I wanted to stay standing up. They were insistent, so I complied. On reflection, I wish I'd been more adamant to give birth in a different position. I had a retained placenta so had to go to surgery after giving birth. The choice of a spinal anaesthetic wasn't given, so I presumed a general anaesthetic was required. I had the same issue with my second child in the UK and was given a spinal anaesthetic. This was much better than a general and I wish this option had been available in Oman. I'm not sure why they insisted on a general anaesthetic for the procedure. We had to stay in for a few days as Isaac was slow to pick up. The care we received during our hospital stay was great (apart from the food!). I think this would probably be the same in the UK. I also feel we might have been out a lot earlier in the UK as they need the beds. I think the few days in hospital gave us some confidence on how to manage our newborn!

Postnatal care doesn't really exist in Oman. In the UK, frequent hospital visits and health visitor visits certainly make the postnatal period easier. In Oman we felt very isolated and very much "left to our own devices", compared to the UK. We sourced private postnatal visits from Karen for several weeks, and I felt these were essential for helping us deal with our new baby. Her guidance and advice were a godsend. The hospitals just didn't offer this service at all.

I think, in summary, I would say using the private system worked well for us and we were fortunate to have the money to afford it. The local system wasn't great for consistency of care and I felt this was important, especially for my first pregnancy. We also accessed private antenatal classes and postnatal services through Karen, as this care wasn't available in Oman. I would advise future expat parents-to-be to investigate the private system where they are, especially if it's their first pregnancy.

What I would do differently:

I would be much more adamant to give birth in the position that I wanted to. I still don't know why the midwives were insistent on me lying on my back, but I feel like this made my birthing experience more uncomfortable than it needed to be. Maybe their training was "old school" and that is the position they want women to give birth in (the midwife staff were all South African rather than Omani, so it surprised me). Only since giving birth in a different position with my second child have I realized how uncomfortable back lying for birth really was.

What I would do the same:

Use the private system. I actually used the same hospital for my second pregnancy, but we were leaving the country before I could give birth there again!

One thing I wish I'd known:

I wish I'd known that general anaesthetics are really not required for placental removal. I would have insisted on a spinal anaesthetic, or would have at least discussed it as an option if I'd known. It was my first child so I just hadn't thought about this as a possible complication post birth.

We now have two amazing children, one born in Oman and one in the UK. I have to say the hospital experience overall was better in Oman.

––––––––

Birth is personal. You are the only one who can give birth to your baby. Sure, you will be in the hospital, under the care of your doctor, midwife and nurses, but you will be the one who is experiencing labour. You cannot control how long your labour will be, or whether your baby will be in the perfect position for birth. You can control your attitude and how you respond to all the events that are occurring.

There are certain things that are out of our control. Certain situations that, despite your best attempts to prevent, may arise, necessitating a change of plan. Let go of what you cannot control. Hold on to what you can. You can control your attitude, your ability to be flexible in the face of unexpected circumstances, and staying connected to your baby, your body and the process of giving birth. You can control your mind, your thoughts, your beliefs and your expectations. Letting go of factors that are out of your control might be a bit daunting at first, but between every event or circumstance that arises and the final outcome, there is a potential space that contains your freedom to choose how you will respond. How you respond greatly influences the outcome and how you feel about the outcome.

Factors out of your control

There are certain environmental, obstetrical, anatomical and fetal issues that are beyond your control.

Environmental factors beyond your control might include a traffic jam that necessitates taking a detour and going to another hospital or weather conditions that prevent you or the doctor from reaching the hospital in time.

Obstetrical issues that are beyond your control might include:

• **Placenta previa** (your placenta covers the cervix partially or completely). This is usually diagnosed by ultrasound during pregnancy, and although you can use visualisation to move it, it may still necessitate a C-section if it remains less than five centimetres from the cervix.

• **Placental abruption** (your placenta separates from the lining of your uterus unexpectedly). This is an emergency and will necessitate an emergency C-section.

• **Cord prolapse** (the cord slides into the vagina ahead of the baby's head). This causes fetal distress and requires an emergency C-section.

• **Post-partum haemorrhage** (your uterus does not contract enough to stop the bleeding after the birth of your baby and your placenta). Your contribution is ensuring high levels of oxytocin during labour and keeping your baby skin to skin after birth. Your baby suckling and nuzzling on your breast, as well as its little feet nudging your belly, all work to release more oxytocin that stimulates contraction. Even so, sometimes this is not enough and you will be given synthetic oxytocin by injection or intravenously.

• **Retained placenta.** This is when your placenta does not separate from the lining of your uterus after your baby is born. If the midwife/doctor is unable to manually remove it, you will need to go to the operating theatre and have it removed under general anaesthetic.

The position of your baby is an anatomical issue beyond your control. There are times when despite staying active during pregnancy and working with the sensations of labour to adapt and change your position during labour, your baby goes into a position that causes a prolonged and difficult labour or into a position that will necessitate a C-section.

Fetal distress is also an issue beyond your control. There are many reasons for fetal distress including position, cord compression, maternal or fetal exhaustion and the influence of medications. Your contribution is to stay connected to your baby, your intuition and the physical sensations of labour that will guide you to move and alter your position to assist your baby during labour and birth. Even so, there are times when your baby gets distressed to a level that requires intervention or a C-section.

Focus on what you can control

The best way to prevent or avoid factors that are out of your control is to focus on the ones that you can control. You can control your mind, including what you put into it and the thoughts you allow yourself to think. Remember what Henry Ford said, "Whether you think you can or you can't - you will be right."

You can control the rate, depth and timing of your breathing. This will take focus that will naturally keep you calm and centred. If your focus is on your breathing, it will be difficult to think negative thoughts.

You can control how much you choose to learn about the process of labour and birth. The more you understand what is happening, the easier it will be to stay out of the negative fear/tension/pain cycle. These are all internal factors that require inner work and practice. They will make the difference in the way that you experience your birth and the way that you remember it.

Christian and Eline Landgraft's birth story, in their own words

In spring 2017 my husband and I decided to move from the Netherlands to Oman because of work. The moment that we agreed to go, was the start of a life-changing rollercoaster. A week after we decided to go, my husband asked me to marry and I was not even used to my wonderful engagement ring when I found out that I was pregnant. Two months later we arrived in Oman to find a house and to find a good feeling for giving birth abroad. I already decided that I wanted to give birth in Oman, flying home and being weeks without my husband and the idea that he should miss the birth was not an option.

I'd read some experiences from expats on the internet and I chose a hospital and a doctor just by feeling. In between searching for a house I visited the doctor and I felt fine with her. I didn't realize that giving birth abroad is not only choosing the right doctor and hospital.

With 20 weeks of pregnancy I settled down in our new house in Oman. My body was changing and I decided to start with pregnancy yoga. Quickly I got in contact with different woman, from all different countries. We shared a lot together, our fears, experiences, our birth plan and preparations. I found out that the way of giving birth is a cultural thing as well. In the Netherlands, where I come from, it is common to give birth at home and nobody talks about pain reduction, we "Dutchies" do it without! We don't even go to a doctor, we give birth with a midwife. Oman was the opposite of what I knew about giving birth. Everything is medical and pain reduction is normal. It is even possible to plan the birth or to choose a C-section. In the Netherlands that is unthinkable.

I believe that the body knows what to do and that the baby knows that as well. I went to the birth preparation course from Karen and there I found the trust that I could have a natural birth in Oman as well, it was all about a good preparation and a good birth plan. My husband and I discussed different scenarios and I wrote my wishes down in a birth plan. I was more than prepared and was just waiting for the first movement.

The day that my water started leaking, I decided to wait a while at home, because I wanted to wait until the contractions started naturally. I knew that when I got to the hospital they would induce me immediate. Unfortunately, the contractions didn't start and I had to go to the hospital. The midwife induced me and after 12 hours the birth started. I went to the labour room and my doctor told me that it wouldn't take long. I was happy to hear that and gathered my last energy together to reach the finish. I decided to use the gas as pain reduction for the last contractions (what I would never have used in my home country). It makes me totally high and I was talking in Dutch and become completely chaotic in my head, but it did reduce the pain! It was a hard fight but my son was still not born and his heartbeat went down. The doctor told me that my son could not come out in a natural way, he was somehow stuck. Before I could realize it, I was in the operating theatre and going under anaesthetic. My husband was standing in the hall and so after all our preparations, wishes and convictions, our son Laurenz got born without his parents in a way what was not in our scenario. A kind of dramatic birth, although I'm so happy that I was in Muscat in a hospital and not in the Netherlands at home. With a home birth we would really have had a challenge because my son had the umbilical cord twice around his neck.

When I look back to my preparations and the choices I've made, I would invest more time in what happens after the birth. I was not well prepared for breastfeeding and that gave me a lot of stress. I was well prepared for the birth, unfortunate not for an emergency C-section. I always believed that children can be born in every place on earth, and actually that is true. In my case, I was really happy that I was in a hospital with a well-prepared team around me. All the cultural differences made me stronger and wiser in making decision and being a mum!

THE ROLE OF INTUITION

Doctors and medical staff do not place much emphasis on intuitive knowing and they do not have much regard when faced with it. I tell you this because it is quite possible that when you start listening to your intuition you may find yourself in a situation where you have to justify it to your doctor or even your partner or family. In doing so you will start to second guess yourself or be talked out of or into something that you intuitively feel is not right for you.

Learning to trust your inner knowing enough to allow it to guide your behaviour, choices and decisions during pregnancy and labour is going to require a lot of practice. You will be faced with many choices and decisions during pregnancy. Some of them will feel wrong and some will feel right. Some will require a lot of research and study. Some will involve opinions from family, friends and professionals. All of them will seem overwhelming at some point or another. This section is about rallying your intuition as a valuable tool that you can rely on.

Intuition is a sense that comes from deep within that just feels right for no apparent reason. Some people refer to it as a sixth sense and others define it as knowing something without prior knowledge. Inner knowing kind of sums all those up for me. Physically, it makes itself known by a fluttering in the belly or a tightness in the chest. When it relates to something that feels wrong, it's like a heaviness, a sinking feeling or a buzzing sound that seems to drown everything else out. When it relates to something that feels right, it's like being held, a feeling of lightness and sense of sureness. It feels almost like being nudged towards or away from something or someone.

I encourage you to create a daily habit of quiet introspection and reflection during pregnancy. This will enable you to tune into yourself, your inner knowing, your inner voice and to your baby. Being able to listen to your intuition requires a deep trust that does not always come naturally, especially when it is juxtaposed with conflicting information, of which there is plenty. There are, however, many ways to use your intuition daily and to practise trusting your inner knowing.

Using your intuition to find solutions

With practice, intuition can give you insight that helps solve a problem or find a solution that you had not thought of previously. Everything you have ever seen, heard and experienced is stored in your subconscious mind. Opening yourself up to your intuition is like giving your subconscious mind permission to access this existing information and find creative ways of problem solving that reflect both reality and experience. What you acquire over time makes your intuition a reliable source of information to make conscious and rational decisions.

Common sense is the capacity to look at the world as it is rather than as it should be, might be, or could be. It reminds us to be aware, attentive and vigilant, and to be patient enough to truly understand a situation before making snap judgements and decisions.

Using intuition to prepare yourself for unexpected news

There are also times when intuition prepares you emotionally for shocking or unexpected news. I have had several of my clients who intuitively knew that they would miscarry. Although this is a common fear among all women, they all told me that it was a strong knowing that moved beyond fear. Of course, this did not make losing their babies any easier, but it helped them to make sense of it of it afterwards and the healing was easier, they said.

It happens just as often with women who know they are pregnant before they have any physical signs. Many women know the moment they conceive. Others have particularly poignant dreams that have significant meaning before or during pregnancy.

Dreams

It is very common to have strange and bizarre dreams when you are pregnant. Dreams are the mind's way of working through daily events, worries and fears. With practice and intention it is possible to ask your intuition for a dream or image that will guide your decision or your behaviour in a specific situation. Allow yourself to be guided by your dreams.

Keep a journal next to your bed so that you can jot everything down as soon as you wake up. Your dreams are vivid and clear in the first moments of waking, but you need to mindfully capture the images and feelings before they disappear. Go to bed with the intention of dreaming about the specific situation or with a specific question in mind. Mentally ask your intuition for a dream or image that will guide your decision in this specific situation. Write or draw whatever comes into your mind immediately upon waking up. Don't worry if you cannot remember the details clearly, focus on how the dream made you feel or any memories it stirred up.

Using your intuition to alert you to take action

Intuition can alert you to take action about something. Like Shirley, who decided to take a five-hour road trip to see her parents when she was 37 weeks pregnant. She had a low-risk, uncomplicated pregnancy and she had a full checkup before leaving and was reassured that all was well with no signs of imminent labour. However, on the second night, she woke up at three in the morning with a strong sense that she needed to get back immediately. Her husband, Paul, did everything he could to convince her to wait until the morning, but despite having absolutely no signs of being in labour, Shirley was adamant that they had to leave that night.

As soon as she was in the car, she relaxed and within three hours she started feeling her contractions coming hard and fast. They headed straight for the hospital and her baby was born within 30 minutes of their arrival. The birth was exactly as she had imagined it and she was so relieved that she had listened to her strong inner knowing. This experience had a deep and lasting effect on her ability to trust her natural instincts to mother her baby.

Intuitively listening to your body

Taking time out to stop and listen, to be in awareness, will help you to shift your focus from the external factors (doctors, hospitals, tests, scans and gadgets) to the internal workings of your mind and body.

So many of the discomforts of pregnancy can be frightening if you take them literally. Your first thought if you experience sharp pain in your lower belly will be of losing your baby. However, you will notice that throughout your pregnancy you will experience many sharp, stabbing and pulling type sensations in your belly, at different times, in response to different things and for different reasons. Most often they are normal. Your labour will also begin with a series of pulling and tightening sensations in your belly, so it is vital that you get used to these new sensations and learn to interpret them. I urge you to use your intuition to tune into these sensations before Googling them.

As you've already learnt in this book, most of the new sensations that you will experience are related to your body's natural safety nets, and usually to the hormone relaxin. I love the word "relaxin" because it reminds one to "relax in" to whatever one is feeling. The moment you experience a new sensation, relax into it. Take a slow and mindful breath and focus your attention on whatever you are feeling:

• Notice where you feel it in your body.
• Describe it to yourself. Is it sharp? Pulling? Stabbing? Tense? Aching?
• Breathe into the sensation and see if you can mentally release it or let it go.
• Ask your inner knowing if this sensation is a normal part of pregnancy or an alert to take action.
• Notice where you feel the answer or how it shows itself to you. Try not to let fear get in the way of your answer or cloud your judgement. Remember that you can always get it checked out to be reassured.

The more you trust your judgement and the more it is confirmed by checking it out, the more you will rely on it.

Using your intuition to connect and communicate with your unborn baby

This is by far my favourite way of working with intuition. I truly believe that connecting and communicating with your baby is easily within your reach and will be one of the most profound experiences of pregnancy. It requires a sense of trust in the way that your baby chooses to communicate with you.

Although it is possible for your partner to do the same, you have the advantage of your baby being inside of you and therefore accessible 24/7. Every aspect of your life, body and experience is affected on some level by the presence of your baby growing within your womb. You are already physically deeply connected, and these exercises will help you to access and strengthen that bond and tap into your, and your baby's, inner knowing.

In the same way that connecting to new sensations will guide you to become more comfortable at understanding and interpreting them, connecting to your baby will guide your actions, choices and decisions during pregnancy and birth.

You and your baby are a team. Your baby does not need to read these books or attend my classes to know when and how to be born. Your body knows when and how to give birth. As you have learnt, labour is a right-brain, primitive activity. It happens largely without your control. It requires a letting go of resistance. Getting out of the way and allowing.

Your baby responds positively to being "seen" and noticed while still in your womb. This appreciation is expressed not only with responsive kicks but also with a feeling of well-being that emanates from your baby and is fed back to you through the invisible pathways of thought and a felt sense of connection in the body.

I encourage you to carve out a few minutes to sit quietly every day, no matter what is going on in your life, to connect with your baby and create your own unique form of communication. This creates a habit of listening and seeing and will give you so much confidence in the first days after your baby is born. You will learn how your baby communicates with you and you will learn to listen to and trust this unique bond that allows you to understand and interpret what your baby needs without words. It will only get stronger day by day and is unique to you and your baby. Nobody will ever know your baby better than you. Ever.

A guided intuition exercise

With your eyes closed, place one hand on your belly and the other on your heart, and bring all your awareness to your breathing.

Notice the gentle rise and fall of your chest with each breath and consciously slow and deepen the breath, noticing that with each breath you become more aware of your body and how you are feeling.

After a few breaths, become aware of your heart beating rhythmically under your hand. Take a moment to enjoy this feeling and then expand your awareness to feel the connection between your heart and your womb, each beat of your heart nurturing your unborn baby.

Feel the natural connection and allow the love to flow, just enjoying this feeling of peace and connection for a few minutes.

Your hands have healing energy. While rubbing your belly imagine healing light or energy coming out from them. Send energy from your hands into your baby. Notice how your baby responds to the loving touch and the thoughts of love and attention that you are placing on him or her.

Think about the things you are grateful for, the love you feel and the love towards this baby, and send it from your heart to your baby.

You may want to add a favourite piece of music to your daily session of connecting to your baby. You could play this at the beginning of each session to relax you and guide you to a place of deep connection, or at the end, as you lie comfortably indulging in the feelings of love and calm. You will be surprised to notice how your baby responds to this piece of music after birth. You can use it when your baby is fussing and you are unsure how to settle him or her. The familiar sounds will soothe and calm both of you and take you back to that place of deep connection. This is an incredibly powerful and beautiful practice.

How does your baby communicate with you?

Your baby can give you a clear idea of what he/she needs in order to feel supported through labour, birth and parenting. Using the same process as above, try and delve a little deeper by getting a sense of what your baby is saying to you. Let go of any expectations or judgements. Engage your imagination and allow yourself to look into your mind's eye, almost as if you are having a dream while in a waking state. When you are in a state of complete relaxation, you may notice symbols, images and colours arising spontaneously.

Allow yourself to get a sense of the energy surrounding your baby. Is it calm? Peaceful? Joyful? Energetic? Mischievous?

How does it make you feel?

What thoughts arise when you pay attention to your baby?

Think of a question and have an imaginary conversation, either quietly in your head or out loud. It does not matter what you talk about, just enjoy sharing your thoughts and notice what thoughts arise for you as you pause to listen. One of my favourite questions is, "What do I need to know before giving birth?" Remember that the answers will not always be literal. They may arise as symbols, images, words, colours or just a feeling.

Acknowledge your baby, be open to what arises and try responding to the messages or thoughts that you receive and notice what happens.

(A recorded version of this meditation is available at www.thevirtualmidwife.com/resources and on The Virtual Midwife podcast on iTunes.)

I encourage you to keep a journal of your thoughts and experiences and when your baby is old enough to open up a discussion when you feel the time is appropriate. I have had many women who have been amazed that their children recall conversations and thoughts that they had while still in the womb, so don't be surprised.

The reason we call intuition our sixth sense is because it is so closely related to our other five senses. The difference, of course, is that the sixth sense is not tangible. Our senses are a protection mechanism. Think about animals who sense a storm coming before there are any visible changes in the weather and retreat to the safety of their basket or a sheltered space if they are in the wild.

In an interaction with someone new, I might *see* that they seem fidgety and nervous, unable to make or maintain eye contact. I might *hear* something that seems incongruent with the situation. I might shake hands and *feel* a cold shiver or a warm touch. These are tangible, noticeable sensations that put my sixth sense into high alert. I use my eyes, ears, hands, skin, emotions, and intellect to capture sensations, information, inspiration, knowledge, and wisdom like a network reaching out to invisible waves of sounds and images. Your senses are decisive factors in the way you manage and make decisions. With a greater awareness of your senses and the data they provide, you will be better equipped to translate your experiences into effective action.

Start listening to your intuition by asking yourself: "If I knew I would receive help from my intuition, what is it I am most concerned about or need to know about this situation?"

Let's assume the situation is deciding where you should give birth. You have visited several hospitals and doctors but you are not fully convinced which one is right for you and your partner. Ask yourself this question constantly while holding the situation in your mind and then allow yourself to observe what is going on without over-analysing it.

This is essentially a "feeling exercise" and you should do it several times and in different states of mind. You might repeat it every time you visit the hospital and see if anything changes. You may find that as you get to know the system better and develop a relationship, you start feeling more positive, trusting, relaxed and open. Or perhaps, the opposite occurs and your inner knowing nudges you to explore other options. You have several months with this particular situation because it is never too late to change your mind, so this is a great one to start with.

• Do you feel anything physically when you think about the situation?

• What is happening in your gut? Your throat? Your chest?

• Does it feel good or bad? Positive or negative? Pushing or pulling?

• Do you get any vivid images in your mind? They could be symbols, shapes or colours or memories of past events. What do these represent for you?

• Do you hear any words or recall past conversations when thinking about the situation?

• What is the overall feeling?

• What are your senses sensing?

• Are your overall feelings and senses congruent with what you have been told or would like to believe?

6. Physical preparation and the stages of labour

Understanding the physical changes in the last trimester and the birthing process

By the time you get to week 35 or 36 you will be feeling heavy, uncomfortable and ready for what has seemed so scary and out of your comfort zone. Your baby is pushing into all your organs, your sleep is disturbed, and you are feeling more pressure over your pubic area and aching in your lower back. You know that this baby cannot get much bigger and you are ready to have your body back. The reality of birth being imminent also starts setting in. If you chose to return home to give birth then you would have had a few weeks to settle and by now you should be clear about your birth choices.

If you haven't already started practising yoga and breathing, then it is not too late and don't delay any longer. Now more than ever it is important that you get connected to the physical changes and new sensations you will be experiencing because every one of them is an indicator of what is going on internally and will guide you to prepare yourself mentally.

Your baby will also start giving you more subtle signs that he or she is getting ready to meet you. You may notice that movement changes or slows down. Remember that there is not that much space to move around anymore, and if the head becomes engaged (meaning that it starts moving into the pelvis) then you will just feel the movements of legs and feet and little wriggles of the body. It may feel completely different to how it did before and can be alarming. As always, check in with your intuition before going to Google.

Whenever you feel that your baby is not moving as much as usual, drink a glass of fresh fruit juice then sit or lie quietly and do a session of connecting to your baby. Go deep and try to get an image of the position your baby is in. Ask your baby for a reassuring sign that all is well. Keep your hands on your belly and your awareness on your hands. Feel the connection between the two of you and tell your baby how excited you are to meet him or her and allow your mind to wander to the day your baby decides to be born. Notice the movement under your hands and count the kicks and wriggles. It is expected that you will feel 10 movements in an hour. However, focus more on the feeling and connection than frantic counting to get to 10.

WHAT IS HAPPENING IN YOUR BODY IN THE LAST TRIMESTER?

Physically and physiologically there are a lot of changes taking place that are absolutely necessary for all your systems to work together harmoniously when labour starts.

The washing machine is a strange metaphor when talking about giving birth, but I am going to use it anyway because it is one that we can all relate to.

When you put your clothes in the washing machine, it is also important to add washing powder, softener, switch the water on, and set the machine on the right cycle. If you forget the washing powder the clothes will get wet but not washed. If you forget the water, they will not be washed at all and the machine will burn out. If you use the wrong cycle the clothes may be washed but not spin and come out all wet. If you add colours to whites, you end up with a wardrobe of pink clothes.

It is exactly the same in labour. There are several things that need to happen internally so that when labour begins, all systems kick into action and work together harmoniously to allow labour to progress normally. All of these things will produce symptoms that can be alarming or reassuring. The better you understand them, the more reassured you will be.

PROBABLE SIGNS OF LABOUR

The following changes are signs that labour is probably on its way, though still not quite here.

Your cervix

Earlier in the book, I talked about your amazing cervix. If you skipped this section then make sure that you read through it before you continue here so that you get the big picture of what happens.

Your cervix will start getting ready to be pulled up by the strong uterine waves or contractions by becoming softer in the last weeks of pregnancy. Medical staff refer to this as ripening.

Although this happens without you realising it, you may feel sudden stabbing pains or needle-sharp sensations in that area. They only last a nanosecond but they are sharp enough to take your breath away and can be quite frightening. Some women experience these more than others, while some don't feel them at all. But if they occur in the last weeks of pregnancy (usually 36 weeks onwards) then it is a reassuring sign that changes are taking place in your cervix. They can be alarming if you do not know what they are, but a reassuring sign when you do.

Sharp shooting pains in your cervix are a *probable sign that labour is imminent* but is not a positive sign that labour has begun.

Your mucus plug

Due to the softening and movement that happens in your cervix, that little plug of mucus that sits at the mouth of the cervix gets disturbed and starts coming away. For some it will come away all at once and you may even hear it drop into the toilet when you are having a pee. Otherwise, you may see streaks of it in your underwear or just notice that you have a lot more sticky white discharge. Streaks of blood, brown or pink, in the mucous would all be considered normal.

Losing your mucus plug is a *probable sign that labour is imminent* but it is not a positive sign that labour has begun. It is merely letting you know that changes are taking place in your cervix, so much so that your mucus plug is coming away. This would be a good time to have lots of sex, making sure that your husband ejaculates inside of you so that his semen, which contains prostaglandins, comes into contact with your cervix, further softening it.

Lower backache

The pressure of your baby moving down into your pelvis will put more and more pressure and strain on your lower back causing an aching, heavy feeling. Once again, this is a *probable sign that labour is imminent* but it is not a positive sign that labour has begun. It is an indication that your baby is moving into position.

Hunger

Very often your body will indicate that labour is probable in the next 24 hours by giving you an insatiable hunger that finds you cleaning out the contents of the fridge and the snack box and still searching for more. It is like carbo-loading for birth.

Although eating and drinking in labour is fine, there is so much going on in your other systems, that the digestive system slows down and you probably won't want to eat. So loading up before is not a bad idea. If you find this happening to you, then go with it. It is a *probable sign that labour is imminent* but it is not a positive sign that labour has begun.

Diarrhoea

This is nature's way of putting your mind at ease that having a poo while you are pushing might NOT happen. The prostaglandins that cause your cervix to soften and shorten in preparation for labour sometimes leak through to your bowel and cause the same softening action that leads to loose stools. This is a great way of emptying your bowels before you go into labour and reducing the chances of there being anything else to push out other than your baby. Loose stools after 39 weeks of pregnancy, especially if coupled with "eat everything in the house", are a *probable sign that labour is imminent,* but not a positive sign that labour has begun.

Braxton Hicks contractions

I refer to these as practice contractions and use the metaphor of going to the gym. The muscles of your uterus need a bit of practice for what they need to achieve during labour and they start "working out" around 25-28 weeks of pregnancy. Most women don't even realise they are having them, and this is why I recommend a regular practice of sitting or lying quietly, with your hands resting on your belly, and connecting to your body and baby.

You will notice sometimes that your belly becomes hard and tight and may even change shape. Often it is caused by your baby moving around, which stimulates the muscles to contract. This is a Braxton Hicks contraction. They last for anything from five to 55 seconds, sometimes even more than that, but they are completely painless. I think that is why they are so difficult to notice and why so many women think that they are not having them. But notice how your belly feels under your hands, and also the shape of the dome. You don't have to experience "pain" in order for it to be a Braxton Hicks, they are more pressure or tightening than pain. They are completely normal and a good sign.

If you compare it to going to the gym it would be the difference between lifting a 1 kg dumbbell and a 10 kg dumbbell. You would easily be able to do at least 10 reps with 1 kg and not feel much in your biceps. So when you are having a Braxton Hicks, your uterus is only doing little contractions, metaphorically equivalent to lifting a 1 kg weight, and they are barely noticeable.

However, once labour begins, the muscles of the uterus need to step up the workout and metaphorically contract to the equivalent of lifting a 10 kg weight. This will be noticeable in the way that you experience it and different in that it continues and a rhythm is established. Remember that this is just an analogy to help you understand the difference between a Braxton Hicks and a labour contraction.

Braxton Hicks contractions are meant to be mild and barely noticeable because we don't actually want them to make any changes to the cervix until your cervix is ready and your baby is ready to be born. If they get too strong too soon then you will go into premature labour. I encourage you to become aware of them so that you can use them as an opportunity to slow down and connect with your baby and use them to practise Directed Breathing. You will learn how to do Directed Breathing later in this chapter, and it is also on my Birth Breathing app available in the Apple App Store.

Working with Braxton Hicks in preparation for labour

Whenever you feel a Braxton Hicks contraction, place your hands on your belly and notice what is happening under your hands. Feel the muscles becoming tense and notice how your belly changes shape and how your baby responds. Move into slow, deep Belly Breathing and focus all your attention on just noticing, feeling and being.

The Braxton Hicks contractions will, therefore, change from being barely noticeable at first to being more noticeable, more frequent and longer lasting after 36 weeks.

How do you know the difference between Braxton Hicks contractions and labour contractions?

The short answer is to change your activity.

If you are resting or sitting quietly when you notice that you are having frequent, noticeable Braxton Hicks contractions, then change your activity. Get up and go for a walk or do a short gentle yoga practice. Do something that takes your mind off the Braxton Hicks for a while and then check in after an hour or two. If they are still there and seem to be getting more frequent and more noticeable then you are probably in early labour. Spend the next few hours balancing resting and getting active, but focus on conserving your energy for when you will need it later in active labour. If you can sleep, then sleep.

If you are walking or doing something physically active when you notice that you are having frequent, noticeable Braxton Hicks, then change your activity. Sit or lie down and put on some of your favourite music. Depending on the time of day, try and have a nap or go to sleep if it is bedtime. Rest for as long as you can without focusing on the Braxton Hicks (if possible) and then check in after an hour or two.

If they are still there and seem to be getting more frequent and more noticeable, then you are probably in early labour and the Braxton Hicks contractions are now real contractions that are regular, rhythmic and steadily increasing in frequency and intensity. Focus on conserving your energy for when you will need it later in active labour. If you can sleep, then sleep. I mean it. I have still not met anybody who managed to have a baby in their sleep, so close your eyes and let sleep happen.

POSITIVE SIGNS OF LABOUR

These changes can be taken as positive indications that labour has finally arrived.

Uterine contractions

These are Braxton Hicks on steroids. They don't go away if you change your activity. They get increasingly more intense and the spaces between them become regular and rhythmic. They are a positive sign that labour has begun. It does not mean you need to go into hospital immediately, but you will become more internally focused and aware of what is happening.

For most women, they will start out as mild, almost unnoticeable, Braxton Hicks and slowly increase in intensity and frequency. Some women don't notice these, though, and so they only become aware of them when they are already quite intense. Either way is OK, but once you become aware of them, you will find that you will need to start using the Deep Breathing technique (refer to the five essential breathing techniques and download the Birth Breathing app) to get through them as they become increasingly more noticeable and intense.

You will not want to talk during a contraction because you will need to focus all your attention on breathing through it. This is what I call the "talk to the hand stage". Breathing deeply through the waves of sensation allows you to stay physically relaxed so the muscles of your uterus can do their job of slowly pulling your cervix up and open. If you tense up when they are trying to do this, your muscles go into spasm and you experience true pain which is hard to move beyond or control with breathing and relaxation.

Regular, rhythmic and strong muscular contractions are essential for your cervix to soften and open and to move your baby out. They are a wonderfully positive and encouraging sign that your baby is getting ready to make the journey to meet you. This is the moment that you have been preparing and waiting for in the last 40 or so weeks. Take a moment to imagine that and notice how it makes you feel.

Your water breaks

This is the rupture of the fluid-filled amniotic sac that surrounds your baby. The pressure within the uterus is stronger at the top (the fundus) to help nudge your baby down and out. If your membranes are still intact (i.e. your waters haven't broken) the pressure from your baby's head on your cervix will be evenly distributed by physics of the amniotic fluid inside the amniotic sac. On the other hand, your membranes may release if your body needs the extra pressure of the baby's head directly on the cervix or the wall of the vaginal passage to help you to bear down.

If you are not having contractions then the breaking of the waters feels like you are having a pee - only it is uncontrollable. For some, it will be a gush, for others a trickle and some of you may actually experience a popping like sensation and possibly even a pop sound! If you are in labour, it will feel like a release of pressure, and there will more than likely be a gush of liquid. After your water breaks when you are in labour, you will experience the contractions and the feeling of your baby pushing down on your cervix differently because the pressure will be increased.

Note that it is not always necessary for the waters to break and it is possible for your baby to be born with the water bag intact. This is absolutely fine. The water bag will break on its own when it needs to, though it is common practice in hospitals for medical staff to suggest breaking your water for you to "speed things up". As with every intervention, use the BRAT method to ascertain if this is the right thing at the right time for you. There are instances where this is necessary and can be used as a useful tool to assess your progress or how your baby is managing, but unless there is a medical indication, it should not be done.

The colour of the fluid when the water breaks is clear, although there may be streaks of pink or bits of blood when it comes out. All of this would be considered normal. If the water is shades of green or brown it could indicate that your baby has had a poo. This could be an indication that your baby is slightly distressed or it could happen if you have gone way over your due date (like 41+ weeks). Although most times the outcome of this is good, it is always a cause for concern and a reason to investigate further. If you are at home and your water is this colour when it breaks, then make your way to the hospital so that they can assess your progress and decide on the next steps. As always, check in with your intuition and stay calm, working with deep breathing.

What if your water breaks and you are not in the hospital and not sure if you are in labour?

There are three things you want to look for if this happens so that you can call your midwife or hospital and tell them the following:

• What colour it is.

• How much (a gush, a trickle, a pool, a tidal wave).

• What you were doing when it happened, for example eating dinner, taking a walk, sleeping, or having sex. By the way, this is a common cause for the water bag to break. The orgasmic contractions of the uterus coupled with the rise in oxytocin and endorphins can be enough to cause the bag to rupture. It is absolutely fine and a great way for labour to start. Do not worry that you have done anything wrong or harmful to your baby. Remember that this is the way your baby started life, so what an awesome way to signal that it is time to meet you. Don't be embarrassed to tell the staff this as it is natural and helps to give us the big picture.

Once the staff have this information they will ask you if you are experiencing any other signs of labour, most noticeably, any contractions. If you are not experiencing any contractions, then it would be better for you to be at home to allow labour to start on its own. If you are experiencing contractions, then you would still be better off staying at home to allow your labour to get into a rhythm.

Be guided by the staff, but remember that once you are in the hospital, they will be resistant to let you go back home, especially if labour is imminent. They will encourage you to come in to be checked out but if nothing is happening (if you are not feeling anything) then it is always better to get labour going in the comfort of your own home where there are no time constraints and you can rest and move about without inhibition. Factor all of these things into your conversation with them and be guided by your intuition rather than fear of something going wrong.

Imagining contractions as waves of sensation

Every time the upper part contracts it causes the lower segment and the cervix to retract or pull up around your baby's head - remember the analogy of pulling a turtleneck sweater over your head? Well, imagine the turtle neck is your cervix and the upper segment is pulling it up and over your baby's head. With every pulling up (of the cervix) there is also a pushing down (of your baby's head on the cervix). This is why I refer to contractions as waves.

UNDERSTANDING PAIN

There are many factors that will influence how you interpret and experience the sensations of labour. Now that you have a clear understanding of what causes the sensations, namely the contractions of the uterine muscles and the pulling up of the cervix, let's look at things that might affect how you perceive these sensations.

Just a little reminder here: the way that you perceive these sensations has nothing at all to do with where you are in the world (at home or in hospital or stuck in a mountain cabin) when it happens. It is how you choose to respond.

Pain vs sensation

Pain is inherently associated with giving birth. There are not too many women who come to my classes expecting an enjoyable birth experience - even though many of them achieve that and it is most definitely possible. However, for as long as you associate pain with labour and use the term pain, it will naturally make you think of unpleasant and abnormal situations like toothache or a broken bone. This pain occurs as a result of something being inherently wrong, and yet everything you will feel in labour is a signal that it is right.

No matter how many people you ask what labour feels like, the answers will fall anywhere on the spectrum of "not nearly as bad as I expected" to "absolutely excruciating", which really does not help you at all because you will naturally focus on the latter.

The fact is that the way YOU experience it is unique, subjective and individual. It is highly dependent on your beliefs and expectations. If you expect it to be excruciating it will be, especially if you are unprepared and afraid. If you expect it to be intense, but you have several powerful techniques that you have been diligently practising, plus you understand that what you are experiencing is an indication that everything is working perfectly, then you will experience it as an intense but challenging experience.

In terms of preparation, think of it this way. If you woke up one morning and decided to run the London marathon, you would have to put a training programme together and prepare. You would never just turn up at the start line with the wrong shoes, no water and no training. You would never consider running a marathon without knowing the route, what to expect, where the hills are or how to pace yourself.

Preparing to have your baby is much the same. By the time your labour begins, you want to be sure that you have done your training and mental preparation. You know the route, (the stages of labour) what to expect, (it's going to be challenging) where the hills are (factors out of your control) and how to pace yourself (rest and conserve your energy during early labour, use deep breathing and "go within" during active labour).

If you have done your training and preparation, then you know that it will be challenging but you also know that you can do it. You will experience sensations of labour, not labour pain. You will know that the sensations you are experiencing are an indication that everything is right and going well. You will have practised tools and techniques to work with the sensations. You know that the sensations are rhythmic and last only 90 seconds. You use your mind and your breath to work with the sensations. You feel prepared and this makes a HUGE difference in the way that you experience and enjoy your labour and birth. Rebecca was prepared. She did not expect to have her baby in the car. She did not expect things to go as quickly as they did. But she was prepared. So when everything happened, it was not scary. She rode the waves of sensation and responded to what her body was doing. She gave birth.

Fear

Fear is a protective mechanism that alerts you to the presence of danger. Fear originates by suggestion or association. As we have already discussed, there is a lot of fear associated with giving birth, especially in the 21st century and the Hollywood dramatisation of birth.

Fear in ordinary, everyday activities makes you look before crossing the road or test the temperature of the bath before stepping in. We do this without thinking. But the fear of labour moves us into an exaggerated sense of caution. How often have you uttered the words "in case anything goes wrong" during your pregnancy?

The fear of pain can actually produce pain through the natural tensing up of muscles in anticipation of the pain. I know that sounds crazy but think about it. If you tense your muscles for an extended period of time, the circulation is affected. Venous blood, which is full of metabolites and waste products, can irritate and lacerate the inner walls of smaller vessels and restrict the free flow of fresh arterial blood. In other words, the persistent tension of the muscles affects the circulation of blood and removal of waste products, which increases the pain in the muscles.

Pain and pressure

It is also important that you learn to differentiate between pain and pressure. The muscles and ligaments in the pelvis are richly supplied with pain and pressure receptors. A receptor is a group of cells that receives stimuli. The contraction of your uterine muscles will produce powerful pressure sensations (stimuli) of birth that may be interpreted as pain, especially if there is tension in the surrounding muscles. In order to manage these sensations, you need to understand how your body processes pain and how your mind perceives it, so here is another one of my analogies.

Imagine the pressure and pain receptors as little cars that carry the impulses to the brain via the spinal cord. Once your labour begins, there is going to be a lot of traffic from the pressure and pain receptors in the muscles of your uterus to your brain via the spinal cord. This means that there would be pressure cars and pain cars travelling to the brain via the spinal cord. There is a little gate between the brain and the spinal cord that they have to pass through. This gate can stop some cars/impulses and allow others to pass through.

Every time your uterine muscles contract and pressure increases there will be stimuli sent to the brain via the spinal cord. If there is tension in the surrounding muscles, it will hinder the ability of the muscle to do its work effectively and this will cause pain. Those little cars just get stuck and the traffic cannot move.

What this means is that you can influence the way you experience the sensation at three sites:

1. The muscles of your uterus where the pain originates:
Practise relaxation techniques to keep your muscles from getting tired and tense and avoid the fear-tension-pain cycle.

Use positions that promote gravity and keep your muscles working in the way they were designed to.

Use deep breathing techniques to keep the muscles well oxygenated and avoid buildup of waste products.

Use deep breathing to stay calm and focused and release tension and resistance.

2. At the gate in the spinal cord:
A pleasant touch stimulus, such as massage or a warm compress, sends positive impulses that can block the transmission of pain impulses through the spinal cord.

You can also cause gridlock at the gate by sending through a lot of competing vehicles, such as impulses from music, specific mental imagery, counter pressure or a TENS machine.

3. In the brain where the pain is perceived:
You can fill up the receptor sites in the brain so that the pain-cars have no place to park. Blocking access to this third pain-perception site is how pain-relieving drugs work.

You can achieve the same effect naturally by manufacturing your body's own painkillers, endorphins, through breathing, relaxation, visualisation, rhythmic movement and support from your partner.

Understanding pressure

There is a vast difference between pressure and pain. Pressure is inevitable as your baby is pressing down on your cervix. Your uterus is pressing down on your baby. Your baby is pressing on all your organs. This pressure causes sensation, but not pain. Close your hand into a tight fist. Notice that there is an increase in pressure, which is a sensation, but it is not painful.

Think about a Braxton Hicks contraction. It is not at all painful because it is caused mainly by increased pressure as your uterine muscles do a little practice run. It happens frequently and unexpectedly and most of the time you are unaware of it.

The accepted belief is that contractions are painful, so that is why you don't notice Braxton Hicks and why many people think they are not "real" contractions. They are real, but they are just caused by pressure and tightening and are not working at full capacity, therefore they are painless. Even so, the way that you experience it has a lot to do with your expected belief that it is NOT painful.

The expected belief about real labour contractions, though, is that they ARE painful. This expectation of pain causes tension in the surrounding muscles which stimulates the pain receptors as well. This creates what we call the fear-tension-pain cycle, which is obviously a negative cycle and definitely not one that you want to be in. This is why deep breathing is so essential because it is impossible to do deep breathing if your muscles are tense.

FEAR = TENSION = PAIN

A reasonable amount of fear of the unknown is normal and expected for all first-time mothers and even second time around. But a deep-seated fear that you are unable to move beyond needs to be addressed during pregnancy, or it will affect your progress in labour. Don't bury them in the hope that they will go away. They will surface as soon as your labour begins and you will move into a negative cycle of fear-tension-pain. If you have not already done so, then go back to the section on fear and do the exercise on reframing and eliminating fear.

The power of suggestion

Unfortunately, medical staff all believe in pain in labour and all suggest, expect and presume pain is present or imminent. I get so frustrated when I have spent hours teaching my clients to work with sensations of labour rather than pain, and the moment they step through the hospital doors, every suggestion, question and comment refers to pain. This suggestion of pain will consciously and unconsciously be conveyed and will be perceived by you through facial expression, actions for relief of "suffering" and preparation for prevention of pain. These are all powerful stimuli for the expectation of and experience of pain.

Comments such as, "Be brave," or, "Don't worry" and questions such as, "How strong are your pains?" all suggest pain and can easily disturb what was previously a peaceful but intense process that you were managing quietly in your own way. As far as possible, try not to be influenced by the ill-timed and inappropriate language used by hospital staff. Change the words in your head and check in with what you are feeling so that you are not affected by suggestions of how you should be feeling.

Often when I worked as a doula, I would arrive at the hospital with a client who was calm and focused, breathing deeply through strong contractions. I would know that she was nearing transition and almost ready to give birth because we had been together for so long at home. However, the medical staff would assume that she was in early labour because of her relaxed manner and apparent absence of pain or fear. On examination they would exclaim in surprise that she was almost ready to give birth and make inappropriate comments, intimating that things were about to get a whole lot worse. The reaction of the hospital staff set up an expectation that did not match the reality of what was actually happening. Had it not been for the deep trust between myself and client, the power of suggestion held the potential to disrupt the calm and positive progress of labour.

Exhaustion

Another factor that will strongly influence the way that you perceive and respond to intense sensations is physical and mental exhaustion. Imagine staying awake and experiencing intense waves of sensation every five minutes for over 24 hours? Even the strongest among you would be exhausted and despondent. It would be easy to just want to give up and give in.

As far as possible, try to get as much rest as you can during the early stages of labour and conserve your energy for when you need it during active labour. Also remember that you are always stronger than you think you are. You will dig deep for resources that you never knew you had in you. That is the beauty of birth.

THE STAGES OF LABOUR IN REAL LIFE

There is a lot of emphasis placed on the stages of labour in books and educational programmes, but although they are relevant and help us (midwives) in our care, it is more important for you to understand what happens in real life! Most of the things you read about don't make much sense at all because a lot of it focuses on how many centimetres dilated your cervix is. The reality is that unless somebody (like a midwife) does an internal examination (also known as a vaginal examination or VE) then you will not know how open your cervix is. I could give you instructions on how to do it yourself but most women don't want to do that and besides, it can be difficult to get your fingers inside when you cannot reach around your belly and even more difficult to interpret what you are feeling.

So although I will go through what happens in each stage, I encourage you to focus on the Labour Cheat Sheet (available at www.thevirtualmidwife.com/resources) which is a summary of everything and will give you a better idea of what to expect to feel, guidelines of what to do with those feelings and recommendations of where you should be.

The idea that there are stages indicates that it is a process that has a beginning, middle and an end. At each stage we expect different things to happen and you cannot move to the next stage until the last one is complete.

Stage 1 labour

BEGINNING (early labour): The cervix starts opening – this is like the warm-up stage. The uterus has started contractions to pull the cervix up and open, but they are still irregular and mild and the spaces between them are long: anything from 10-30 minutes apart.

MIDDLE (active labour): The cervix is actively opening – there is a rhythm to the contractions, anything from three to five minutes apart. They are regular, more intense and requiring your focused attention to keep working harmoniously to open your cervix.

END (transition): The cervix opens fully and the baby is moving into position to be born. Your uterus changes function so that it is now only pushing down onto your baby, so this is often the most intense time as you feel increased pressure to push.

Stage 2 birth

In the second stage, your baby is pushed through your fully open cervix, into your vagina and is born.

Stage 3 birth of placenta

In the third stage, the placenta comes away from the wall of the uterus and is pushed out of the vagina.

You will not necessarily know what stage you are in most of the time and it does not really matter. Your job is to BE. You do not need to DO anything because your body does it for you. The contractions are involuntary. All you need to do is to let go. Let it happen. Feel it and don't fight it.

BREATHING TECHNIQUES FOR LABOUR

It might seem strange that you need to learn specific breathing techniques when breathing is such a natural, everyday thing that we do without thinking. At any given moment, you are intimately connected to your breath and yet we don't take much notice of it. There is no other time when you will experience such intense physical and deep emotional changes than when you are giving birth. There is no doubt that your breathing will change depth, pace and rate as you experience the physical sensations of labour.

Think about how you respond when you hear bad news – that sudden intake of breath and then a slowing down of your breathing as you take the news in. Think about how you respond when you are afraid, the way your breath becomes shallow and fast. Think about how your breathing changes when you are making love. You won't always be aware of the change in depth and pace of your breathing because it occurs in response to physical and emotional changes in your body and is largely subconscious. So you definitely want to be aware of your breath and have some well-practised techniques that you can turn to when you feel like you are losing control. Your breath is like your lifeline during labour and birth. These exercises will help you to take notice of your habits and learn powerful techniques to cope with the intensity of the sensations.

Each of these breathing techniques is important in its own way and should be practised with awareness during pregnancy. They all work together, and although I encourage you to go through them individually and become comfortable with each one before moving on, you will soon move through them all seamlessly together. The more you practise them the more natural and instinctive they will become, just as it is during pleasure and arousal.

What you are working towards is a deep awareness of the power of your breath to guide and transform your experience. You know that labour and birth will be a physically challenging event. By practising these techniques daily in different situations and with expanded awareness, you will instinctively move into these breathing patterns when you need them, with gentle guidance from your partner.

THE FIVE ESSENTIAL BREATHING TECHNIQUES

I recommend that you download the Birth Breathing app for iPhone and use it to practise the five essential breathing techniques for labour. The app includes instructions and a timer to do a daily practice and check in the resource section.

1. Easy Breathing

Easy Breathing is the easiest one, but in many ways the most important one. You will use Easy Breathing in the space *between contractions*. That might sound strange because all other techniques are used *during contractions*. However, if you are unable to relax *between* contractions, then relaxing *during* contractions will be virtually impossible. So they are both extremely important.

How to do it right now

Close your eyes and bring your awareness to your breath. Just notice it. Start by noticing if you breathe IN through your mouth or your nose and what feels comfortable. Then notice if you breathe OUT through your mouth or your nose and what feels comfortable.

There is no right or wrong with this one so just keep breathing with all your awareness on both the in-breath and the out-breath. Notice the feel of the cool air in your nostrils. Notice the gentle rise and fall of your chest. Notice the rate of your breathing. Notice the depth of the breath - or how far it extends down your torso. Don't make any attempt to change anything, just notice and breathe. See if you can do that for two minutes without your attention wondering off. Keep bringing your attention back to the breath if you notice it wandering off.

How to practise it on a daily basis

Whenever you get in the car to drive somewhere, spend a minute before starting the car taking notice of your breath. Let it be smooth, calm and effortless. Do this several times a day during normal daily activities. Notice how difficult it is to bring your awareness to your breath and keep your awareness on your breath for more than a minute. I am certain it will be a struggle initially, so persevere. It seems mindless, but it is a vital skill in labour.

How to do it in labour

Easy Breathing will be more difficult during labour because there is so much more going on. Your partner needs to be aware of this exercise and its importance so that he can watch and guide you to relax between waves and make sure that your breathing is smooth and effortless, as you prepare mentally for the next wave of sensation. The point of Easy Breathing is that it is easy. Effortless. Relaxing.

Easy Breathing is an awareness of allowing your breath to be smooth and effortless. It is more of an awareness than something you actively do.

You will use it in the spaces BETWEEN contractions in labour.

2. Deep Breathing

You will use Deep Breathing during every contraction/wave of sensation that you use during labour. Deep Breathing will *keep you focused* and will provide a form of distraction. By consciously Deep Breathing you will easily be able to stay relaxed during the natural contraction of the uterine muscles, allowing them to do the work of drawing up and opening your cervix. Notice that when you do this breathing, it is virtually impossible to breathe deeply if any or all of your muscles are tense. So this is an excellent way of learning to LET GO of any tension or resistance.

How to use it during labour
In the beginning of your labour, the sensations will be more of a tightening and not at all painful - more like longer and stronger Braxton Hicks contractions. As your labour becomes more established and rhythmic you will notice that the sensation becomes more noticeable, lasts longer and the time between them becomes more regular. You will find that you do not want to speak during a wave and you will naturally turn your attention more inwards and become more focused. This is when you need to breathe slowly and mindfully, focusing on releasing tension with every exhalation. As soon as the contraction passes, slip back into effortless Easy Breathing.

How to do it right now
Make sure that your shoulders are completely relaxed by rolling them around a few times and allowing them to drop down away from the ears. Practice deep breathing by inhaling through the nose to the count of two seconds and exhaling through your mouth to the count of four seconds. This means that each breath is a total of six seconds. Make sure that that your shoulders don't move up at all. You should feel the breath moving through your nostrils and then feel your chest rising and your ribcage expanding as your lungs become fuller with each count. Take your time. Focus on inhaling slowly for two seconds and then slowly exhaling for four seconds.

How to practise it on a daily basis
Use the demonstration app to time your breathing. Set the timer of the app for two minutes so that you can focus fully on nothing but slow and deep breathing. Notice the sound and feel of the breath and the physical movements of your body.

In summary, Deep Breathing is slow and mindful and keeps you focused. Practise it when you find yourself panicking or in stressful daily situations. Use it DURING contractions in labour.

3. Belly Breathing

Belly Breathing is very similar to deep breathing. The pace of Belly Breathing is the same as Deep Breathing with an in-breath of two seconds and an out-breath of four seconds - the difference is in the depth of the breathing. With Belly Breathing you will feel the breath moving all the way down to your belly and your belly moving out as you breathe in. Imagine you are using your breath to blow up a balloon in your belly. Every breath in fills the balloon and every breath out empties it.

You will notice when your baby is born, that this is how babies breathe naturally. This is actually how we are meant to breathe, but over time, our breathing becomes shallow and less effective. I encourage you to practice this daily from 15 weeks until the day you give birth with conscious attention.

Belly Breathing helps to strengthen the abdominal muscles and brings a deep awareness to your body. Your baby also loves it and you will no doubt notice that he or she starts moving and squirming about in your belly each time you practice this.

How to do it right now
Start off by doing the exercise when you are seated and place your hands on your belly. Inhale slowly through your nose to the count of two, and exhale through your mouth to the count of four. Feel the breath moving through your nostrils, notice your chest rising, your ribcage expanding and your belly slowly filling and moving outwards towards your hands. Take your time, don't rush this. Use the feel of your hands on your belly as your guide - this is what you are breathing into and you should feel your belly expanding outwards towards your hands on the inhalation. Gently draw your belly in as you exhale. Imagine the breath moving up and out of your mouth. Try and make a soft sighing H sound as you breathe out to the count of four, feeling your belly moving inwards towards your spine. You will need to actively draw the abdominal muscles inwards, almost as if you are pulling your tummy in to zip up your jeans. Do it slowly and mindfully, imagining that you are gradually squeezing the air out of the balloon with your belly.

How to practise it on a daily basis
In stage 1 you are sitting comfortably in your chair. In stage 2 you will need to be on your hands and knees in an all-fours position. Spend a few days practising in a seated position. When you feel confident that you know what you are doing, move to stage 2 on your hands and knees. I urge you to practise this daily until the day you give birth. You will notice how challenging it becomes to practise it on your hands and knees as your belly gets bigger. It is a great way to tone and strengthen the abdominal muscles without doing any harmful core exercises. Set your intention to do it for at least five minutes every day.

How to use it during labour

You can use Belly Breathing in the exact same way as you would use Deep Breathing in labour. The pace is the same but the depth of breathing is different. Use what feels most comfortable to you. Belly Breathing is more important in pregnancy than in labour. If you have practised it daily then you will naturally default to using Belly Breathing and this will feel comfortable for you. If you find that Belly Breathing takes too much effort and concentration during labour then use Deep Breathing.

The most important benefit of breathing is to *keep you focused* and provide a form of *distraction*. By consciously breathing you will easily be able to stay relaxed during the natural contraction of the uterine muscles, allowing them to do the work of drawing up and opening your cervix. Notice that when you do this breathing, it is virtually impossible to breathe deeply if any or all of your muscles are tense. So this is an excellent way of learning to *let go* of any tension or resistance.

In the beginning of your labour, the sensations will be more of a tightening and not at all painful – more like longer and stronger Braxton Hicks contractions. As your labour becomes more established and rhythmic you will notice that the sensation becomes more noticeable, lasts longer and the time between them becomes more regular. You will find that you do not want to speak during a wave and you will naturally turn your attention more inwards and become more focused on your baby, your body and your breath.

In summary, Belly Breathing is slow and mindful and keeps you focused. It is very similar to deep breathing, but your breath and awareness extend to your belly.

Practice this during *pregnancy* - your baby will love it and it strengthens your abdominal muscles, especially when practised on your hands and knees.

Use it during contractions in *labour* - but only if it is effortless. Otherwise, use Deep Breathing.

4. Directed Breathing

Directed Breathing is a combination of elements from Deep Breathing and Belly Breathing with an expanded internal focus and awareness. It is about applying the same techniques but to different areas of your body. In many ways it is more of a mind exercise. You are using your mind to guide your breath to a specific area in your body and giving your mind clear instructions what to do with each breath. Directed Breathing is an invaluable tool for managing the pain of a contraction, and it will also assist the dilation of the cervix as you direct your breath to relax and expand in the pelvic region. It is a great tool for relaxing and reducing tension anywhere in your body and mind. It is easy, effortless, sustainable and relaxing. You can modify it as you adjust to the changes in the labour process.

How to do it right now
Close your eyes and place your hand on your chest. Bring your awareness to the feel of your hand and mentally direct your breath into your hand as you feel your chest expand. Imagine exhaling from this area while you intentionally relax the area under the hand and in your chest. Do not move the hand until you are able to intentionally expand each area with your inhalation and relax each area with your exhalation. Once you have mastered an area, move your hands to a different area on your body.

Partner practice
When you are working with your partner, one of you will be the *doer*, or the person placing hands. The other will be the *receiver* or the person taking at least three breath cycles to deeply expand and relax into the doer's hands. Play around with it, placing your hands in different areas of each other's bodies and working together to create breath awareness and interchanging between being the doer and the receiver.

Try the same exercises with the receiver in different positions: standing, lying, or kneeling. Notice how the same spots soften/relax better or not so well depending on body position. Pay attention to which positions create the deepest expansion and relaxation.

Fast forward a moment in time to see yourself in labour and to imagine how this gentle support of your partner's loving touch will be able to help you through the uncomfortable sensations.

How to practise it on a daily basis
There will be endless opportunities to practise this daily. Every time you get a strange pain or pulling sensation, a wave of nausea, a mild headache or lower backache. Every time you experience a new or different or uncomfortable sensation is an opportunity to practise Directed Breathing.

Start by becoming aware of the sensation, where you are feeling it and what you are experiencing. Is it tightness, pulling, hurting, throbbing or a dull ache? Now direct your breath to the sensation. Direct your mind to release the sensation with every out-breath. As you breathe out, imagine letting it go, see and feel it becoming smaller and less noticeable. Keep doing that until the sensation goes completely or becomes more comfortable as you relax the muscles and area surrounding it.

How to use it in labour

Directed Breathing is an incredibly powerful tool to use in labour when you are well practised at releasing tension and sensation with your mind and breath.

You can use it to:

• release muscle tension and resistance during surges, making them more effective and more comfortable for you

• mentally dilate the cervix by directing the mind to imagine expansion in the area where you are feeling pressure and intense sensation

• feel the support and love through your partner's touch and use it to keep yourself calm and focused

In summary, Directed Breathing is still Deep Breathing but it engages your mind to direct your breath to where you feel tension or discomfort. Practise this during *pregnancy* whenever you feel a strange or uncomfortable sensation. Use it during *labour* to release tension anywhere in your body or just to be aware of your partners loving touch.

5. Birth Breath

The Birth Breath is a combination of Deep Breathing to pace you, Belly Breathing to utilise the abdominal muscles on the exhalation, and Directed Breathing to focus the mind. It is as much a *mind* technique as a *breathing* technique and it's important that you visualise what is happening as you feel it.

It might sound strange to compare having a baby with having a poo but the concept is very similar and it will help you to practise this technique so that when you are ready to give birth, it will be easy to use.

When your body digests food, the waste products are moved gradually down the intestine until they reach the rectum and are passed through the anus. They are moved by a process called peristalsis. This is an involuntary constriction and relaxation of the muscles of the intestine which creates wavelike movements that push the contents of the intestines forward.

When the contents reach the end of the canal they exert pressure on the nerve endings that send a signal to your brain that lets you know you need to go to the loo. The *involuntary* peristaltic waves continue but now that you are on the loo, you couple that with the *voluntary* effort of bearing down or pushing so that you can eliminate the waste products in the loo.

When your baby is ready to be born, the baby is moved gradually down from the uterus, through the dilated cervix and through the vagina to be born.

The baby is moved by involuntary constriction and relaxation of the muscles of the uterus which creates wavelike movements, called contractions, that push the baby forward. When the baby reaches the end of the vagina (which is directly in front of the anus and rectum) it exerts pressure on the nerve endings that send a signal to your brain that lets you know you need to give birth. This feeling is exactly the same as the feeling to have a poo, only much stronger. The *involuntary* contractions continue but now you couple that with the *voluntary* effort of bearing down or pushing so that you can give birth.

Have a poo and having a baby are a combination of *involuntary and voluntary* bodily functions. Having a poo is a combination of *involuntary peristaltic* waves coupled with *voluntary bearing down*. Giving birth is a combination of *involuntary uterine* waves coupled with *voluntary bearing down*.

Understanding this principle means that you are able to mentally practise and visualise every time you go to the loo. Every day when you go to the loo to have a poo there is an opportunity to practise this breath. If you are battling with constipation during pregnancy, then this is going to help you a lot! It will take a bit of practice to get it right, but you will know when you do. Keep practising it so that you commit the sensation to cellular memory.

How to practise it on a daily basis

Every day when you go to the bathroom, make sure that you sit on the toilet with your shoulders relaxed, hands resting in your lap.

Bring all your awareness to the feeling of pressure in your rectum and around the vagina that is caused by the pressure of your stool.

Close your eyes and start slow deep breathing, extending the exhale to a slow count of four or even five.

Focus all your attention on the out-breath and direct it to the feeling of pressure.

Every out-breath is an opportunity to relax, release and let go of the pressure.

Allow your body to relax completely as you direct your breath and your mind to releasing.

You may or may not feel the contents of your bowel moving down slowly aided by the peristaltic waves. If you do not feel it, then imagine it. If you do feel it then keep releasing with exhalation. Remember that your stool is being moved down by the *involuntary* contraction of your bowel and you are just aiding that with your breath and your mind.

At some stage of this process you may feel an urge to voluntarily push or bear down to move things along. If this is instinctive then go with it. After all, you have never taken so much notice of the process of having a poo and it is very much an automatic behaviour.

Practice this every day, noticing how much easier it becomes to direct your breath to your bottom and direct your mind to release, relax and let go. Notice how little effort it can take when you allow the involuntary peristaltic waves to do their work, supported by your voluntary effort of Directed Breathing and ultimately bearing down effectively.

How to use it in labour

You will use this technique towards the end of your labour when you feel pressure around your vagina and rectum and it feels like you want to make a massive poo. This is caused by the pressure of your baby's head pressing down on all the nerves and pressure receptors in that region. The Birth Breath is a powerful and extremely effective breathing technique to help you navigate this challenging stage before you are about to give birth. If you have practised during pregnancy, you will instinctively move into this type of breathing when you feel your baby pushing down on the same area in the moments before birth.

By practising this breath, your focus will be on letting go. Letting go of the natural inclination to "hold it in", letting go of resistance to the intense sensation, letting go of inhibition, letting go of your fear that you are about to give birth, letting go of the subconscious desire to keep your baby safe inside of you and last, but not least, letting go of your "old life" to become a mother.

Benefits of the Birth Breath:

• You will avoid "purple pushing".

• You will not need to be coached (people shouting "push, push!") because you will be guided by the power of your surges.

• You will be working with your baby – real teamwork.

• You will feel more in control.

• You will protect your pelvic floor by not over straining with purple pushing.

• You will decrease the need for an episiotomy.

• The slow gentle movement of your baby down the vagina will allow slow stretching, which means that tearing is unlikely and avoidable.

In summary, the Birth Breath is a combination of deep breathing to *pace* you, Belly Breathing to utilise the abdominal muscles on the exhalation, and Directed Breathing to *focus* the mind.

It is as much a mind technique as a breathing technique and important that you visualise what is happening as you feel it.

Practise this during *pregnancy* every time you have a poo.

Use it during *labour* when you start feeling intense pressure to push.

PUSHING AND BIRTH

So often, women will feedback to me that they did not know how to push or that they were told that they were doing it wrong. I am always dismayed when I hear these stories because, as awful as it seems, pushing a baby is so similar to having a poo. Nobody has ever told you that you are doing it wrong and I am certain that you know exactly what you are doing when you go to the toilet every day. There is never any second guessing yourself of wondering if you are doing it correctly. You just feel an urge to go to the bathroom to have a poo, you sit on the loo and you do it. In saying that, it would not be so easy if you sat on the loo trying to have poo without having any urge to do so. I mean you could sit there for hours, push until you are blue in the face and still nothing would happen.

Your pelvic colon, rectum and anus are directly behind your cervix and vagina. As your baby moves down the birth canal, you will start feeling more intense pressure and an irresistible urge to bear, similar to wanting to go to the toilet. If you do not feel this pressure and urge then it means that your baby is still high. Your cervix may be open but your baby is still moving down and it is just a matter of time until you start feeling pressure to push.

In hospitals where there are sometimes unnecessary time constraints and pressure to get things over with you may be encouraged to push before you have the natural urge to push. It would feel the same as trying to have a poo without needing to have a poo. Just sitting on the toilet and pushing and pushing and hoping that something comes out. This is called purple pushing and wherever possible you should avoid it. It is exhausting for you and your baby and will damage your pelvic floor due to the increased pressure and exertion of pushing against nothing.

How to avoid purple pushing
Do not push unless you have the urge to push.

What if the staff are telling me that I am ready to push?
In this case, you would want to know if they are wanting you to push because there is a problem. Please note that if this situation occurs, then it will most likely be after many hours of labour and you and your partner will be tired and ready to go with whatever is being suggested. It is not the ideal time for negotiation and questioning and I recommend that your partner takes the lead here as you will be "in the zone" and you do not want something like this to get you out of the zone. In fact, as far as possible, you need to keep focusing on what is happening to you while your partner asks the following questions:
• Are you concerned about the baby? Is there any sign of fetal distress?
• Is there any immediate/urgent reason to encourage pushing now?
• Can we delay pushing until my partner feels the urge to push and, if so, will you give us the time and space to allow this to happen without interruption? You can add that you have done significant preparation for your birth and that you understand how important it is that your partner is able to work with the natural urge to push. You understand that the baby needs to move into the best position for this to happen. You might use this time to work together with your partner to change positions to encourage your baby to move down. Any position that opens the outlet of the pelvis will be good here, so consider a forward-leaning wide-knee child's pose or a deep partner-supported squat.

When your baby reaches your vagina it will exert pressure on the nerve endings that send a signal to your brain that lets you know you need to push. Your uterus will also change function and actually start pushing down, making your natural urge to push even stronger. Start actively using the Birth Breath. If you have been practising this daily when you go to the toilet, then you will instinctively move into this type of breathing when you feel your baby pushing down on the same area in the moments before birth. The Birth Breath is a combination of Deep Breathing (to pace you), Belly Breathing (to utilise the abdominal muscles on the exhalation) and Directed Breathing (to focus the mind).

It is as much a mind technique as a breathing technique and important that you visualise what is happening as you feel it. Regardless of what position you are in, direct your focus to where you feel the pressure and direct your mind to work with your body to release, relax and let go until the urge is so overwhelming that you engage your abdominal muscles to bear down more effectively. Your passive pushing has now become active bearing down and you will soon meet your baby.

The precious moments after birth
Wherever possible, and in most hospitals, it is standard practice for your baby to be placed directly onto your chest after birth. At this stage your baby is still attached to you via the umbilical cord and the placenta and is still receiving blood from the placenta. The first few moments are miraculous in so many ways. You are meeting your baby for the first time, hearing the first cry and your baby is taking his or her first breath. While all this is happening, the entire circulation system of your baby is changing as the lungs begin working.

It is beneficial for you and your baby to spend the first minutes after birth completely uninterrupted. This includes not clamping or cutting the umbilical cord until it has stopped pulsing. This allows most of the blood that is in the placenta to pass through to your baby. This blood is rich in oxygen, nutrients and stem cells that are vital for your baby's long-term health. Unless there is a valid medical reason to cut the cord immediately after birth, it is always recommended to wait at least five minutes, which is usually how long it takes for all the blood in the placenta to be transferred to your baby.

There are two viewpoints that need to be considered at this crucial time:

From your viewpoint, it is a moment of absolute bliss and relief. Your body is flooded with the hormone oxytocin and you are literally falling in love while taking in the enormity of what you have just achieved. You need time to take it all in, stroking your baby's soft skin, smelling your baby, feeling your baby moving on your chest, listening to the cries and whimpers, and feeling your instinctive maternal responses kicking in. All of these emotions augment your oxytocin levels which naturally helps your placenta to separate.

From the viewpoint of the hospital staff, you and your baby are safe and well and time is money. The sooner they can get the placenta out, clean you up and get you back to the ward, the better. This sounds incredibly harsh and inhumane, but it is the reality of clinical practice. In a busy hospital, the precious moments after birth are not honoured as they should or could be. The emphasis is on good clinical outcomes.

Ideally, you would like both. Good clinical outcomes AND unhurried and uninterrupted contact with your baby during which time your placenta will naturally separate anything between five and 30 minutes after birth. We call this a natural physiological third stage.

The alternative to physiological third stage is to actively manage the birth of your placenta. You will be given an injection of Syntocinon or Syntometrine at the top of your thigh just as your baby is being born or soon afterwards. This injection causes strong uterine contractions that stimulate the placenta to separate quicker. Usually the doctor or midwife will use gentle, controlled cord traction to help the placenta out. It may feel weird but it is not painful as the placenta is soft and much smaller than your baby.

I highly recommend discussing this with your doctor or midwife during your 38-week check-up when you talk about your birth wishes. Remember to use the BRAT method to guide your discussion and talk about the importance of five minutes of unhurried and uninterrupted skin to skin contact.

If this is not possible for some reason then it is not too late to do it later. Skin to skin contact is important for the first few weeks, not just the first few moments after birth. Always remember that it is your intention that counts. In the event of something happening that prevents you from having this time immediately after birth, you can still stay emotionally connected to your baby in exactly the same way that you have done throughout your pregnancy. Do not sever this invisible deep connection and move into fear and anxiety. Allow the feelings of love and support to be conveyed to your baby through this incredibly powerful bond that you already have. Even if your baby is not in your arms and skin to skin, you are still intimately connected.

Physical touch is important but emotional connection is essential.

7. Navigating common hospital interventions

How to make informed decisions about the various treatments and interventions you will be offered

Earlier I talked about the safety nets of pregnancy and how your body naturally does things to keep you and your baby safe. While they are natural and expected, they can be represented as a *problem* and in an effort to *solve* the problem, an intervention is recommended.

You are entering uncharted territory when you go into the hospital environment and this is even more challenging if you are in a foreign healthcare system. This is why I place so much emphasis on trust. You need to trust what is happening in your body. You need to trust that your partner has "got your back". You need to trust that your care provider understands you and respects your wishes. You need to trust that the hospital caters to your specific needs and treats you with dignity and respect as a birthing woman.

If you want to avoid unnecessary interventions it is essential that you know why they do them and what questions to ask so that you can be sure it is the right choice for your situation. Unfortunately, there is a lot of fear-mongering from the people you have placed your trust in. Hospitals are more interested in safe outcomes than warm, fuzzy experiences. You, however, want both, and there is no reason why you should not get both. The harsh reality is that you will need to be proactive in your communication, and you will need to understand enough about common interventions to be able to weigh up the risk/benefit ratio in each situation.

Unfortunately, it is impossible to predict in advance exactly what may happen during your labour and birth, or how a given intervention may affect you or your baby. While it is never the intention of any intervention to cause harm, it is important to accept that many maternity care interventions have unintended effects. They may or may not have the intended effect, and sometimes they have unplanned and unwanted effects. These effects are new problems that need to be addressed with further intervention. We call this the cascade of interventions.

There is a fine line between interventions that prevent unexpected complications and those that can lead to complications in a normal physiological labour that is progressing well. Commonly occurring practices that can lead to further intervention include:
• induction of labour without any medical indications
• AROM (artificial rupture of the membranes) surrounding the baby before or during labour augmenting a naturally progressing labour with synthetic oxytocin (Syntocin or Pitocin) to make labour move faster
• giving medications for pain relief when not requested by you, with a full understanding of the risk/benefit ratio
• being confined to bed during labour versus being upright and moving about

In many cases, these practices cause problems because they disrupt the normal physiology of pregnancy, labour and birth by:
• interfering with oxytocin and endorphins that move labour and birth along and help you to cope with the intensity of the sensations and physical challenge
• increasing the opportunities for infection (for you and your baby)
• causing fetal distress
• making it harder for you to push your baby out
• increasing pressure on you to "perform" according to hospital protocols and expected norms

The key to navigating interventions lies in being able to look at the bigger picture. Remember that nothing can be treated in isolation. This is especially true in labour and birth. Whenever a decision is required you want to make sure that you have all the relevant information and then engage in a conversation with the staff to make a decision that works for both of you. Key elements of decision making include clarifying that there is a decision to make, identifying the options, presenting pros and cons of the options and helping you think about how the options might align with your values and preferences.
• What stage of labour are you in?
• What is the situation we are dealing with?
• Was labour progressing normally until now? What changed?
• What are we trying to achieve?
• What is the best-case scenario? Could we achieve this with watchful waiting or is an intervention necessary?
• How far off the "expected norm" am I at the moment? Could this change?

Making informed decisions

Regardless of where you choose to give birth, or what country you are in, you will need to take responsibility for making informed decisions about your care. It is your legal right to give permission or to deny permission for your care and that of your baby. It sometimes means having the courage and confidence to ask tough questions of potential or current care providers and birth setting staff to ensure the options you want are available to you.

You may feel uncertain or uneasy about becoming so actively involved in decision making but studies have shown that most women are interested in a detailed account of possible benefits and harms before accepting a specific course of action, and so you should be.

Maternity care providers are responsible for meeting the legal standard of informed consent. This means that providers must tell you about the possible benefits and harms that a reasonable person in your situation would want to know to make an informed decision.

Informed consent

Informed consent is not always a form or a signature. It is a process between you and your care provider that helps you decide what will and will not be done to your body. A vaginal examination is a common procedure that is done in almost every maternity case at some stage of the labour. A vaginal examination is invasive and embarrassing for many women. It makes you feel incredibly vulnerable and you need to be relaxed for the midwife to be able to do a full assessment. It is vital that she takes the time to tell you why she is doing it, how it is done, what she hopes to find out from the examination and if there are any risks to performing it at this stage. You have every right to decline the procedure and your healthcare provider is responsible for explaining:
• why the medical procedure, drug, test or other treatment is being offered
what it would involve
• the harms and benefits that are associated with this medical procedure, drug, test or other treatment
alternatives to this care, and the harms and benefits of those other options, including the possibility of doing nothing other than watchful waiting

The purpose of informed consent is to respect your right to self-determination and autonomy. You have a right to clear and full explanations about your care and answers to any questions you may have. It can be hard to have these conversations in a busy healthcare setting with so much going on, but it's important to set aside the time to discuss these issues with your care provider, both in advance and when it is time to make a decision. If at any point during pregnancy, these conversations raise concerns that your maternity care provider or your planned birth setting is not a good match for your values and preferences, you may want to explore other options. Do not be afraid to seek a second opinion or even to change your care provider. Your doctor is not your friend. You are paying them for a service and you will not offend them by changing. In fact, they will probably not notice, and if they do, perhaps they should have been nicer.
Key phrases and open-ended questions to help you:
• I don't understand (situation/intervention).
• Please explain this (situation/intervention) to me more clearly.
• What could happen to me or my baby if I do or do not do what you are suggesting?
• What if I take no action, otherwise known as watchful waiting? Is this safe in my situation?
• Would you care to share some research to support what you're recommending?
• Do I have time to gather more information before making my decision?
• I have some information I'd like to share with you.
• I'm uncomfortable with what you are recommending. What are my other options?
• I'm not ready to make a decision yet.
• I'm thinking about getting a second opinion.

Tatiana's birth story in her own words

I arrived in Oman when I was already four months pregnant. My husband had been there for longer already and he only brought me over when he had settled into his job and found our house. We had lived in other countries as expats before so luckily I was good at connecting with local meetup groups. The pregnancy care that I had in Russia was amazing and I had my own midwife who I wanted to bring with me to Oman, but it was just not possible. I was planning to return to Russia to give birth with her.

Then luckily I met Karen and she helped me to find good prenatal care. I loved her yoga classes and met another pregnant lady who is now one of my closest friends, even though we are again separated because I have since moved to Germany with my husband. I had always been low risk but towards the end of my pregnancy, my doctor informed us that our baby was not growing fast enough. Medically this is called IUGR or intra-uterine growth retardation, which sounds so awful. I wanted to return to Russia immediately but the doctor would not give me the necessary approval for the flight and the airlines would not let me fly without it. When I got to 34 weeks they suggested that I have an induction as she was still not growing and staying any longer would put her health at risk. I was terrified. We went for a second and even a third opinion and all the doctors said the same.

Karen helped us a lot by telling us what questions to ask and making sure that they gave us alternatives but by the time we had seen these doctors we knew that having an induction, even with all its risks, was the best plan for us. As Karen said, the benefits outweighed the risks in our situation. She also helped with some visualisation exercises. I knew that I wanted to have a natural birth and that having an induction increased my chances of having a C-section or other interventions. I do not know if the visualisation helped or not, but my labour started within hours of the first tablet that they inserted and progressed really fast. Our daughter was born weighing 2.78 kg but perfectly healthy. She did not even have to go into the NICU as they had warned she may have to.

Informed refusal

If you disagree with your care provider and decide not to accept care, you have a right to informed refusal. Even if you signed a form agreeing to a particular type of care, you have the right to change your mind.

Evidence-based maternity care

Evidence-based maternity care means using results of the best research about the safety and effectiveness of specific tests, treatments and other interventions to help you make decisions about your maternity care. While healthcare systems strive to ensure that the care they provide reflects the best available research, they are busy and it is hard to keep up with and understand the large and ever-growing body of research on any given maternity topic.

Even when they understand lessons from the best available research, it can be hard to change established beliefs and routines and even policies of care. This is why it's important for you to take time to understand the quality of evidence and what has been shown to be beneficial or harmful. Some basic principles of evidence-based healthcare are to question common assumptions and to ask for evidence:

Question common assumptions: Be sceptical! Many widely held beliefs about healthcare do not reflect the best available research. This may lead to poor care and poor health outcomes. A classic example of this is immediate cord clamping. The research clearly shows that it is beneficial to wait until the cord has stopped pulsing before clamping and cutting the cord, and yet in many hospitals the policies have not yet changed accordingly.

Ask for evidence: When available, well-conducted systematic reviews of research should inform care decisions. This focus on high-quality evidence helps support your informed decision making. With this in mind, let's go through some of the common interventions that are done in hospitals so that you can get a deeper understanding of why they are done when they are necessary or not necessary. How to avoid them and how to negotiate them during labour.

Please download the BRAT Pack from www.thevirtualmidwife.com/resources where I have outlined the benefits, risks, alternatives and timing of each of the following interventions.

Intravenous (IV) therapy in labour

If you opt to have a hospital birth, you will most likely be faced with the choice to either consent or deny the placement of an intravenous catheter or IV. This is inserted into a vein in your hand or arm and will either be hooked up to some fluid, like normal saline, or closed off with a little cap called a saline lock or hep lock. Once you have the hep lock in, it can be used to give you fluids or to administer medications.

Medications administered via IV are instantly absorbed into the body, making it ideal for quick results and also to keep you hydrated in the event that you do not want to eat or drink, or have been told not to eat or drink. This sometimes happens in hospital situations where they prefer you to keep an empty stomach in the event of needing an emergency C-section under general anaesthesia. Since labour and birth are not medical emergencies and if your labour is progressing normally then it is usually advisable to wait until the need for an IV actually arises. Unnecessary placement means unnecessary risk.

Induction of labour

I haven't met many pregnant women who are not totally over being pregnant by the time they reach 38+ weeks. I love watching the journey as they start attending my prenatal yoga classes in early pregnancy and glance enviously around at the bigger bellies. They sigh when they hear the other moms talking about feeling kicks and punches and they count the days until they finally feel those first flutters. They can't wait to look really pregnant. Fast forward 30 or so weeks and they are feeling tired, uncomfortable and heavy and ready to say yes to any possibility of having their baby sooner. Although there are medical reasons for inducing a labour, being tired of being pregnant isn't one of them.

An induction of labour is a series of interventions that attempt to mimic or replace the natural processes that happen during the last weeks of pregnancy in order to speed up the process dramatically. Induction of labour techniques work on your cervix, your contractions, your membranes and your hormones.

For example, in an induced labour, your cervix is artificially softened using prostaglandin gel or tablets that are inserted into your cervix. The prostaglandin is left for 8-12 hours to start working, during which time you will be monitored. If nothing happens then they may repeat the dose and wait another 8-12 hours and then decide what to do next, depending on how your cervix has responded and whether contractions have begun. Remember that once the process has started, it must continue. The tablet is trying to achieve in a few hours what normally takes weeks.

When is induction medically indicated?

There are several medical indications for induction of labour. If you do not have any of these then an induction is not necessarily the right choice for you and you will need to have the BRAT conversation with your care provider.

1. Post dates: Your estimated due date (EDD) falls around the 40-week mark. Many hospitals have a policy of induction at 10 days after the EDD. Various studies have compared induction of labour at or after 41 weeks with watchful waiting that involves repeated tests of fetal wellbeing between 41 and 42 weeks. Check the policy at the hospital you have chosen so that you are prepared to discuss the BRAT if your pregnancy goes beyond the 41-week mark.

2. PROM (premature rupture of membranes): Traditionally, PROM before 37 weeks without labour starting spontaneously within 24 hours would be seen as reason for induction of labour. However, eight studies with a combined total of 1 230 babies of women with ruptured membranes between 34 and 37 weeks of pregnancy found no advantages for induction compared with waiting for labour with respect to C-section or infection or breathing problems in babies.

3. Suspected large baby: There is no accurate way to measure a baby's size and weight before birth, so babies are only "suspected" to be large until they are born.

4. IUGR (intra-uterine growth retardation) at term: A diagnosis of IUGR relies on accurate dating in early pregnancy and regular follow-up throughout pregnancy. Ultrasounds are more accurate before 20 weeks, when the margin of error is 7-10 days. Ultrasound dating at or near term is more likely to have a margin of error of three weeks.

5. Oligohydramnios (significantly decreased amniotic fluid): The amount of fluid can be measured during an ultrasound to ascertain the AFI or amniotic fluid index. If the AFI shows a fluid level of less than five centimetres, the absence of a fluid pocket 2-3 cm in depth, or a fluid volume of less than 500 ml at 32-36 weeks gestation, then oligohydramnios is suspected.

6. Pre-eclampsia or PIH (pregnancy induced hypertension): This can be extremely dangerous to both you and your baby. If your blood pressure shoots up slowly or suddenly during later pregnancy, they will try to stabilise and treat it, but you may be offered an induction or C-section depending on the severity.

Augmentation of labour

Augmentation of labour is the process of stimulating the uterus to increase the frequency, duration and intensity of contractions. It is different to an induction in that it happens only after spontaneous labour has begun, and only in the event that it slows down significantly or is not progressing as expected. The contractions are stimulated with the use of intravenous oxytocin infusion (also called Syntocin or Pitocin) and/or the artificial rupture of your membranes, AROM.

Prolonged labour, often called failure to progress, has become one of the leading causes of unnecessary C-sections, particularly in first-time mothers.

Rupturing of membranes (breaking of the waters)

In the movies, labour always begins with a dramatic version of the water breaking, usually in a public place and everybody going into a state of panic. The baby is born soon after, without any sign of labour between the event and reaching the hospital OR by the time she reaches the hospital, both she and her baby are in grave danger and they are miraculously saved by the fast-acting ER staff. In real life, there are four ways that your water bag or membranes might break:

• SROM (spontaneous rupture of membranes): Your membranes release on their own (spontaneous) at term once your labour has begun. Term is anywhere between 37 and 42 complete weeks.

• PROM (premature rupture of membranes): Your membranes release on their own (spontaneous) before labour begins.

• PPROM (preterm, premature rupture of membranes): Your membranes release on their own (spontaneous) before 37 weeks gestation.

• AROM (artificial rupture of membranes): Your membranes are ruptured by your health care provider to induce or accelerate your labour.

Why is AROM done?
• to stimulate contractions to start labour (induction)
• to strengthen contractions to prevent prolonged labour
• to regulate contractions in a labour which has stalled or not progressed
• to introduce monitoring devices, such as a fetal scalp electrode or an intrauterine pressure gauge
• to assess the fetal condition by checking for the presence of meconium liquor

Even though the idea of shortening your labour may sound fabulous, if it requires interventions then there are always trade-offs that you need to be aware of. Once an ARM is performed, your labour is closely monitored and you will be on time limits. You may also be advised to have continuous electronic foetal monitoring. Many women report labour as being more difficult following artificial rupture of membranes, requiring pain relief.

You should not be put under any pressure to commit to having your waters artificially broken in order to receive pain medication, gain access to the delivery suites, or to avoid routine interventions. It is essential that your verbal consent is obtained to perform an AROM.

What the evidence says

Evidence does not support artificial rupture of membranes for women in normally progressing spontaneous labours or where a woman's labour has become prolonged. In 15 studies involving 5 583 women, the evidence showed no shortening of the length of the first stage of labour and a possible increase in caesarean section. Routine AROM is not recommended as part of standard labour management and care.

Medical pain relief options

Even if you go into labour with a plan to avoid medication, it is good to know that there is always a safety net of medical options available to you, and you can change your mind at any time. This section will give you an understanding of how they work, how to weigh up the risk-benefit ratio and when the best window of opportunity is for using them.

Entonox

This is a mixture of oxygen and nitrous oxide and is sometimes called laughing gas. It is not always available so check with your hospital during pregnancy so that you know if it will be in case you need it. You breathe it in through a mask or mouthpiece which you hold yourself.

TENS machine

TENS stands for transcutaneous electrical nerve stimulation. Electrodes are taped onto your back and connected by wires to a small battery-powered stimulator known as an obstetric pulsar. Holding the pulsar, you give yourself small, safe amounts of current which sends pleasure signals to your brain. Pleasure signals travel faster than pain signals, so your brain is stimulated to produce endorphins.

Pethidine/statol

Injections of drugs like pethidine can help you relax, and this can make labour contractions more effective because there is no resistance. It is administered by intramuscular injection in any major muscle group like your bicep, thigh or buttock.

It takes 20 minutes to feel the effects and will last for 4-6 hours. Your midwife will do a vaginal examination before giving you pethidine. Given too early, it can stall your labour as it is a strong muscle relaxant so there needs to be a good rhythm of contractions. Given too late, it may speed your labour up and your baby may be born still feeling the effects of the drug and may have problems breathing. If this happens, there is an antidote available which will be given to your baby to reverse the effects of the drug.

Epidural

An epidural is a special type of local anaesthesia that numbs the nerves which carry pain from the pelvic area to the brain. For most women, an epidural gives complete pain relief. It does, however, remove all sensation so it means that movement is limited. You will not be a proactive participant in your birth as much as before because you are now very much high risk and will need to be closely monitored. An epidural given to a low-risk woman with a labour that is progressing normally can very easily lead to the cascade of interventions I spoke about earlier. An epidural can be very helpful for women who are having a particularly long labour or who are becoming very distressed.

Episiotomy and perineal tears

Wherever possible you want to avoid these and give birth with an intact vagina and perineum. Learning to use the Birth Breath (see the five essential breathing techniques) is essential as this will help you to move your baby down slowly and gently and in your own time.

Perineal massage started at 35 weeks and done twice a week will reduce the chances of having an episiotomy during birth. You will need to get your partner to do it for you because you probably will not be able to reach down there. He will need to insert one or two fingers into the vagina and apply downward and sweeping pressure towards the perineum, gently stretching the perineal tissue. Use a lubricant to make it more comfortable and use it as an exploratory form of foreplay.

Once you are in labour and nearing the second stage, do not rush to push your baby out. Try not to be pressured to move things along any quicker than what is happening naturally. The pushing and birth stage is the culmination of many hours of labour. It signifies the end of your pregnancy journey and the beginning of your motherhood journey. You will more than likely be feeling exhausted and you will have to dig deep to find the resources within to keep going. Now more than ever is the time to connect with what you are feeling in your body and with your baby, and work together as a team.

What is an episiotomy?

A cut made in the area between the vagina and anus to widen the opening of the vagina, allowing the baby to come through it more easily. The National Institute for Health and Care Excellence (NICE) recommends that an episiotomy should be considered if the baby is in distress and needs to be born quickly or if there is a clinical need, such as a delivery that needs forceps or ventouse, or a risk of a tear to the anus.

These are the only two reasons that an episiotomy should be considered and you should always give your verbal consent if it is required.

How to avoid it

I highly recommend speaking to your doctor and midwife at your 38-week checkup. During this conversation you want to be reassured that they will support your wish to avoid an episiotomy with the understanding that you have done considerable preparation yourself (breathing exercises, perineal awareness and perineal massage) and that you will be using specific breathing techniques during labour to allow your baby to move slowly and the perineum to stretch adequately. You need to know that they will support you during this process and not pressure you to push harder or faster than is necessary. It goes without saying that this would be in the absence of any of the two indications for an episiotomy.

Will they use local anaesthetic?

Another thing that I highly recommend to avoid having an episiotomy is to not allow them to give you a local anaesthetic into your perineum while you are pushing. Very often this is done "just in case" you need an episiotomy and sold to you as being better because you will not feel it if it needs to be done. The truth is that you will not feel it anyway, even without the local anaesthetic. I know that seems hard to imagine, but there will already be so much sensation down there, so much stretching and burning, that any release (whether it is because your baby's head emerges or because the skin tears or the skin is cut) will feel like a relief.

A local injection into the area where all your attention is focused is counterproductive. You will not be able to feel anymore and it will affect your ability to work with the pressure of your baby's head. It will also decrease the ability of your skin to stretch because the interstitial spaces have been filled with fluid. In my experience, as soon as the local injection has been given, it will be followed soon afterwards by an episiotomy. By declining the local, you will increase your chances of not having one and if you do have one or if you have a tear, they WILL give you a local before doing the suture repair.

Recovery after an episiotomy

The cut or tear will be sutured with material that dissolves within 10-14 days. It will take two to three weeks until you feel normal again. Use sanitary pads that have been soaked in a mixture of water with a few drops of witch hazel and then frozen, for relief. Place the frozen pad into your underwear and a towel under your bottom. The cool pad reduces swelling and the witch hazel has healing properties. As soon as the pad starts thawing, clean the area well with another bit of cotton soaked in witch hazel and then put a clean dry pad in place. Use the frozen pads 3-4 times a day for the first few days and then as needed. Make sure that you eat a diet high in fibre so that your stools are soft and regular and drink plenty of fluids.

ASSISTED BIRTH

Sometimes, even when you have done everything you can to give birth with minimal interventions, you might reach a point where you need a bit of help. This could be because your baby is not moving down and out as would normally be expected, despite your effort. Or it could be because there are concerns about your baby's well-being during the pushing stage (fetal distress).

The purpose of an assisted vaginal birth is to mimic a normal vaginal birth with minimum risk to you and your baby. This means that along with your pushing efforts, your doctor will use instruments (ventouse or forceps) to help your baby to be born.

There are two methods of assisted birth and your doctor will usually decide in the moment which one is the best, depending on your circumstances and why your baby is not moving down as expected.

Ventouse

A ventouse is a small suction cup that is attached to your baby's head and used to give gentle downward traction while you are pushing. Very often this is used if your baby's chin is not tucked in enough. Remember the analogy of pulling a turtleneck sweater over your head? Well, imagine trying to put the sweater on by placing the opening on your forehead instead of your crown. Your forehead would be the presenting part and you would be pulling it over your face. We naturally tuck the chin into the chest to position the opening over the crown and then apply downward traction to pull it over the head. So the purpose of the ventouse cup is to assist your baby's head into a more tucked in position by placing the cup on the crown and giving downward traction. If this is done at the same time as your pushing efforts and the downward pressure of your uterus then it will help your baby to move out of your vagina easier with the crown as the presenting part rather than the forehead.

Forceps

Forceps are smooth metal instruments that look like large spoons or tongs. They are curved to fit around your baby's head. The forceps are carefully positioned around your baby's head and your doctor will gently pull and guide your baby out while you are pushing. Forceps are sometimes used to try to turn your baby into the correct position, for example, if your baby has its back to your back in the late stage of labour. Remember that positioning and movement during labour can help you to move your baby into the correct position, so make sure that you stay active and work with your body. Although ventouse and forceps are both safe and effective, they both carry risks that are better avoided wherever possible. Assisted vaginal birth is less likely to be successful if:

- your baby is large

- your baby is lying with its back to your back or posterior position

- your baby's head is not low down in the birth canal

Having an assisted vaginal birth does not mean you will necessarily have one in your next pregnancy. Most women who have an assisted vaginal birth deliver spontaneously next time around. Even if your assisted vaginal birth was performed in theatre, you have an 80% chance of having a spontaneous birth next time. If your doctor is not sure whether your baby can be safely born vaginally, you may be moved to the operating theatre so that you can have a caesarean section.

Caesarean section

For most of you, this is not the preferred option, but I urge you to stay open to things not always going as expected. Plan and prepare for what you want, but not to the exclusion of what you don't want. Remember that a C-section is a birth option and one that can potentially save you and your baby from a traumatic birth or prevent a poor outcome. If you know and understand why and when a C-section may be necessary then you can do your bit to prevent it, with the understanding that there are certain factors that are out of your control, that could lead to requiring a C-section.

Let's start by going through the factors that are within your control that will influence the likelihood of you needing a C-section. I have purposefully indicated whether these choices are made during pregnancy or once you are in labour as there is a big difference. During pregnancy you still have time to plan and change your mind, change your doctor, change your hospital or even change your country. However, once you are in labour, your choices are limited by the care provider and the policies and practices of the birth setting you are in. In the event of being faced with the decision to have a C-section, it is highly unlikely that you can change your doctor or move to another hospital. This is why the questioning techniques and discussions are so important during pregnancy so that you are able to gain a sense of trust in your choices and know that they are the right ones for you.

DURING PREGNANCY: Your choice of care provider and birth setting
I know that many of you reading this are expats and you may feel as if your choices are limited. Perhaps they are, but if this is your reality then make the best of a bad choice and make sure that you are well prepared and informed to be proactive in your care.

C-section rates vary from less than 10% for some care providers and birth settings to more than 60% for others due to differences in policies and practices. It depends a lot on how they support you in labour, in their judgment about when to recommend surgical birth and in their comfort level with variations from the norm and ability to cope with routine complications.

In my experience, even when you ask a doctor or hospital what their C-section rates are, the answer is irrelevant. The WHO recommends a C-section rate of no more than 15 percent of normal labour. The reality is that most hospitals are running at 40-60 percent and they will justify it by saying that the birth outcomes are good. But you and I want a good birth outcome AND a good birth experience. So you want to be sure that the doctor and place of birth that you choose will support both of these wishes.

DURING LABOUR: Your access to supportive care during labour
Support during labour can be provided by your husband or partner, or you can choose to hire a doula. A doula is a woman who is trained to attend to your emotional and physical needs during labour and birth and will be with you continuously. She does not have any medical training, but she understands the physiology of labour and her role is to support you through the intensity of the process. Having a doula with you is becoming increasingly popular and increasingly necessary because of the general state of health worldwide. There is an acute shortage of well-trained midwives and this means that it is highly likely that although you will have a midwife at your birth, she will quite possibly be attending you and several other women at the same time. She will not be able to provide continuous support to all of you at the same time. This is not ideal for you or for the midwife, but in many cases it is the reality.

A doula fills this gap by having the necessary training and experience to give you the one to one care and attention that you need. I cannot recommend hiring a doula enough, especially if you are in a foreign environment. A lot of research has been done on the benefit of having trained continuous support and it has been proven that women who receive continuous support are more likely to have spontaneous vaginal births and less likely to have any pain medication, epidurals, negative feelings about childbirth, vacuum or forceps-assisted births, and C-sections.

Although your husband or partner is the person you most want with you, admittedly he is not trained in support measures and does not necessarily know the hospital system or what is best.

Having a doula present gives your partner the space and confidence to be the best support he can be for you, by knowing that there is someone else who has your back. A doula can be your advocate and your sounding board.

DURING LABOUR: The medical interventions you experience while giving birth

As mentioned earlier, there is a fine line between interventions that prevent unexpected complications and those that can lead to complications in a normal physiological labour that is progressing well. Commonly occurring practices that can lead to further intervention include:
• induction of labour without any medical indications
• AROM before or during labour
• augmenting a naturally progressing labour with synthetic oxytocin (Syntocin or Pitocin) to make labour move faster
• giving medications for pain relief when not requested by you, with a full understanding of the risk/benefit ratio
• being confined to bed during labour versus being upright and moving about

In many cases, these practices cause problems because they disrupt the normal physiology of pregnancy, labour and birth by:
• interfering with hormones oxytocin and endorphins that move labour and birth along and help you to cope with the intensity of the sensations and physical challenge
• increasing the opportunities for infection (for you and your baby)
• possible undesirable effects on your baby causing fetal distress
• making it harder for you to push your baby out
• increasing pressure on you to "perform" according to hospital protocols and expected norms

Let's look at a classic example of a cascade of interventions. Way back when I was working in a busy L&D ward, I would often come into contact with women who went into labour with the intention of having an epidural for pain relief. When epidurals first came into fashion they were extremely popular. Everyone wanted one. Their decision was based the belief that an epidural would mean a "painless" and therefore a "good" birth. Most often they had not done any research or reading on the benefits or risks and if they had, they still felt that the benefit of removing all pain far outweighed the risks of the epidural. Although an epidural does indeed provide complete and very effective pain relief, it has many risks that need to be considered when deciding that this is a good option for you:
• The medication used increases the risk of experiencing a sudden drop in blood pressure which will require IV fluid, which may cause a fluid overload.
• An epidural may cause a longer labour or labour may slow down in which case you will be given Syntocin/Pitocin to augment your contractions and get things going again.
• The epidural drugs or the drugs used to augment your labour may cause your baby to be distressed.
An epidural is a medical procedure and you will require continuous fetal monitoring as you will not be able to feel the contractions and we do not know how you will respond to the drugs used.
• An epidural causes loss of sensation and often function from above the waist down. You will be confined to bed and unable to move into favourable positions to help your baby down and out.
• You will need a catheter as you will not be able to feel when your bladder is full, which will impact your baby's ability to move down.
• You may not be able to feel to push your baby out - this may require forceps or vacuum to help the baby out.
• You may feel disconnected from your baby as your physical sensation has been numbed.
• You may get a fever which may make doctors worry that your baby has a fever, so your baby will have blood tests and possibly antibiotics after birth or be kept under observation. This means they will be apart from you, which will impact your bonding and breastfeeding.
• The drugs used can cause itching, which will require more drugs to control, and which will be passed to your baby in utero.
If you take all of these factors and potential risks into account in a labour that is progressing normally, meaning that there is constant change and progress, then having an epidural would just be opening up to a host of other interventions and complications that could be avoided.

Non-medical reasons for a C-section

There are some of you who may choose to have a C-section rather than giving birth vaginally. I believe that you should always have a choice. After all, it is your body. However, I will always give you all the information and full disclosure and make sure that we have gone through all the alternatives before supporting your choice to have an elective C-section.

I have met several women over the years with an extreme and profound fear of childbirth. While almost all pregnant women are fearful about giving birth, this level of fear is much greater. Sometimes it stems from a history of sexual abuse but it can just as easily be from a particular story or image that has stuck in their mind. For these women, the fear of giving birth is so extreme that it will ultimately get in the way of them being able to go into labour or allow it to progress spontaneously purely because of the fear/tension/pain syndrome. They also do not see any benefit for themselves or the baby of being born vaginally. The only thing that matters is getting the baby out without having to go through labour and birth. To be able to schedule abdominal surgery is infinitely more appealing than this, and the recovery period associated with surgery is preferable to the challenges of birth. If this rings true for you then seek counselling with a therapist who has both strong counselling skills and an understanding of maternity issues. Be sure to talk this over with your care provider as early as possible in your pregnancy, and work together to help ensure the safest and most satisfying birth possible.

There is also a rising trend to schedule a C-section purely for convenience and speed, and also even according to specific astrology dates. Although this may sound appealing and despite taking a lot go the guesswork out of it, it is not recommended in the absence of any medical indications. A C-section is major abdominal surgery and has its own risks and benefits to you and your baby. It is important to weigh these up when making your decision and to consider how important the birth is for both you and your baby.

Medical indications for a C-section during pregnancy

There are some conditions that are recognised during pregnancy that will preclude you from being able to give birth vaginally:
• Placenta previa: Your placenta is lying close or completely covering your cervix which means that your baby cannot be born vaginally.
• Breech position: Your baby is positioned head down or even feet down. This is not an absolute indication for C-section and babies can be born vaginally in the breech position, but you will need to find a care provider who has the necessary training and expertise to be with you for a breech birth.
• Twins or multiple pregnancy: As with breech, this is not an absolute indication for C-section, however multiple pregnancies are treated as high risk.
• Transverse lie: Your baby is lying across your belly and will not be able to be born vaginally in this position. Unless your baby changes position, you will need a C-section. Very often this is due to an abnormally shaped uterus and will be identified by ultrasound scan.
• Previous C-section within two years: Once again, this is not an absolute indication and will depend very much on your particular circumstances and decided in discussion with your care provider. It is advised to wait at least two years before falling pregnant after a C-section if you want to have a vaginal birth the next time.

Medical indications for a C-section during labour

1. Prolonged labour: Your labour is taking a long time often referred to as "prolonged labour" or "failure to progress". This is a tricky one because labour is meant to take long and every woman labours in her own time. This is why choosing your care provider and birth setting is important, as they will vary in how they might try to prevent or respond to a slow labour, and in their patience with a long labour. Some will try to rest the uterus, make suggestions of position changes or encourage you to spend some time in warm water. Some will suggest augmenting your labour, stimulating stronger contractions with drugs before recommending a C-section. Others will be quicker to turn to a C-section immediately. As long as you and your baby are doing well, there is no medical reason to get a C-section, but bear in mind that if you have reached this point, you will be feeling exhausted and desperate yourself and a C-section may be a very appealing option. Having a doula can help you get through a long and challenging labour and guide you about the options available. An experienced doula will support your partner and help them help you.

2. Changes in the fetal heart rate: When your baby's heart rate is very fast, very slow or irregular, your care provider may be concerned that there is some form of distress and that getting your baby out quicker is the safest option. As always, we need to look at the bigger picture. What stage of labour are you in and are there any other signs of distress. In some situations, the heart rate can be improved by moving to another position or by giving drugs to stop contractions. If these strategies don't work and the baby is not about to be born, a C-section may be recommended. Electronic fetal monitoring (EFM) can falsely suggest that the baby is in trouble, so further testing may be required.

3. Prolonged second stage: This is when you have got all the way to being fully dilated and you are already pushing but, for some reason, your baby is not coming down. If you have been actively pushing for more than one hour with no progress, there will usually be a discussion about assisting your birth, either with ventouse or by going for a C-section. It is very disappointing when this happens, although often it can be a relief because by this stage you will be exhausted. There is also a possibility that there is some fetal distress due to the prolonged pushing which would impact the decision to go for a C-section.

Remember that if a decision to do a C-section is made while you are in labour, it will be called an emergency C-section, even if there is no true emergency. There will be time to discuss options and decide what is best for you, your partner and your baby before signing the consent and going ahead.

In a true emergency, where either you or your baby, or both of you, are in grave danger, the decision will be made in haste and in an atmosphere of urgency. The staff will be moving fast, the emergency bell or alarm will be rung and everyone will swing into action to get you into the operating theatre as quickly as possible while preparing you and getting you to sign consent. There will be no time for discussion and you will be very aware that this is an emergency that requires quick action.

Absolute indication for C-section – true emergency

1. Cord prolapse: This is when the umbilical cord comes out before your baby's head and there is cord compression in the vagina every time your uterus contracts. The risk of this happening is 0.1-0.6% and slightly higher than 1% if your baby is in breech position. It is diagnosed during a vaginal examination and can only happen after your water has broken. You will be prepared for immediate emergency C-section as it is not possible to push the cord back up or past your baby's head.

2. Uterine rupture: This is usually a complication of a previous C-section where there is a weakness along the scar tissue that is under pressure during labour. It is a true emergency. The incidence of uterine rupture with no previous surgery is 0.87%. If you have had one prior vaginal birth after C-section the risk reduces to 0.45% and again to 0.38% with two prior VBC.

3. Placenta abruption: This is when the placenta separates from the lining of the uterus before your baby is born. The placenta is your baby's lifeline so this is a grave and serious complication that requires immediate surgery to get your baby out. The incidence of placental abruption occurring is 1%.

There are always times when a normal labour does not progress as expected and you will be advised to have a C-section. This is always disappointing, especially if you have put considerable effort into preparing yourself for a vaginal birth. This is the time when you have to let go of how you imagined it might be and go with what is happening. Most often it will be due to reasons that are out of your control, a bit like rain on your wedding day. It wasn't in the plan, it meant you had to make a few changes and maybe your hair got ruined, but you still got married and it was still a memorable day – more so because of the last-minute changes.

Epilogue

I watched Rebecca's confidence flourish as her pregnancy progressed. She diligently attended my prenatal yoga classes and connected with other like-minded women in class. At that stage my classes were predominantly expats and they bonded over their shared experience of feeling flung way out of their comfort zones and isolated from their family back home during this special time in their lives. They made up for it with the adult version of playdates, making the most of the bounty of freedom they had during the day, and planning extended shopping trips to Dubai to browse and buy baby clothes and equipment. Rebecca and Jason threw themselves wholeheartedly into preparing for a natural birth in one of the private hospitals in Oman.

I guided them gently through the system and supported them when they changed doctors not once but three times until they found one they felt comfortable with. I coached them through the various communication techniques described in this book and agreed to attend the birth with them as their doula. (Although I am a midwife, the rules in Oman do not allow an outside midwife to attend a hospital birth for medico-legal reasons. By calling myself a doula, I was able to attend as a support partner with the understanding that I was not allowed to perform any medical procedures.)

Rebecca's labour started at home at around 5 a.m. I encouraged them to try and get some more sleep and they managed a few hours until I got a call again at 10 to say that things were picking up. I packed my "doula bag" that consisted of a tennis ball in a sock, (the best thing for some deep back massage) some lavender essential oil, a cooler bag with some cold towelettes and a few healthy snacks in case any of us got hungry. I had a flashback when I arrived at their house, recalling the day not even nine months before, that Rebecca and I sat facing each other, sitting in deckchairs, her sobs echoing in the empty room. This time, Rebecca was smiling and radiant. "Its happening," she said, rubbing her hands over the expanse of her belly. Jason stood proudly next to her, pen and paper in his hand, reading out the timing of the contractions for the past hour. I could see that we still had a fair while to go and what we needed more than anything was distraction. "Let's have a cup of tea," I ventured.

"But shouldn't we go to the hospital?" asked Jason.

"We will. but not yet. We don't want to be there too soon." I reminded them about hospital timelines and the need to be in an established labour pattern to minimise unnecessary interventions.

"Right, yes, absolutely," he said, and Rebecca moaned her agreement as the first contraction she had since I arrived swept over her.

I started loud Deep Breathing, establishing eye contact with her and indicating for her to breathe along with me. I watched as her body softened, her eyes closed and she breathed through the sensation. We breathed and walked and talked and drank tea for another four hours before I started quietly suggesting that it was time to move to the hospital. The car was already packed and Rebecca was deep in the zone, completely focused on her breathing and the sensations of labour. She found it too uncomfortable to sit in the front seat so she knelt on the back seat, facing backwards. The only thing she said the during the journey to the hospital was, "Turn that off!" when Jason slipped her favourite CD in, thinking it would be a good distraction.

It took us almost 10 minutes to walk from the car to the labour room as Rebecca needed to stop every few minutes to breathe through her contractions. I could see that she was near and was glad we had made the call to move to the hospital. The midwife who examined her was shocked that she was almost fully dilated and called for a wheelchair. The look on Rebecca's face was comical.

"I will NOT get into a wheelchair!"

"But it's hospital policy," the midwife countered.

"I walked into the hospital, I can walk to the labour room," she said, quietly but firmly. Then she turned and waddled slowly out of the room, only to stop a few steps later to breathe loudly through her next contraction.

"Wow!" I thought. Where was the quiet and timid Rebecca I had met that day in the empty lounge? This woman was powerful. Protective. On fire. I felt so proud of her.

The midwife rolled her eyes at me, pushing past Jason as she gathered up her notes and then leading the way to the labour room. She set about getting the delivery pack out and ready and I heard her calling Rebecca's doctor and saying, "She's almost fully dilated and she will go quickly. I hope you are nearby."

Rebecca just kept doing her thing. She pulled her clothes off and started fanning herself. I could see she was in transition.

"Not long to go now, my love," I whispered and she nodded. She was pacing the room, making low grunting noises. The midwife wanted her on the bed. I warned her off with my eyes, knowing that she would find her way to the bed when she needed to. Ten minutes later she did. Jason helped her up, supporting her from behind as she let out a deep guttural roar. I saw his eyes widen in horror, looking at me questioningly. I smiled back, reassuring him that this was not only normal but fantastic. A moment later she reached down between her legs to feel the tufts of hair as her baby emerged. The midwife was scrambling frantically to get her trolley ready and the doctor had just walked into the room, but Rebecca was totally in control and was not waiting for anyone. The doctor stepped forward, gently coaching her and guiding her baby out.

Barely 45 minutes after walking into the hospital, Rebecca and Jason welcomed their baby girl gently into the world. Swathes of dark hair and a perfectly pink rosebud mouth opened in a healthy cry to signal to the world that she had arrived. This precious baby girl. Made in New Zealand - born in Oman. With love and trust all the way, just like every baby should be born, regardless of whether it is in a hospital bed, a cottage in the mountains, a rice paddy or the back of a car. Love and trust were present when your baby was conceived. Allow it to be present when your baby is born.

An invitation

I have been supporting expat families around the globe for over a decade. As a midwife, I understand what your care provider is talking about. I know that it's often hard to understand what doctors and nurses are talking about so I will prepare you ahead of time and can translate in the moment.

The *Virtual Midwife Programme* is a sequential journey designed to give you the confidence to get the right care at the right time and includes essential tools and techniques required when giving birth in a foreign healthcare system. It requires a commitment of time and effort, but the results are life-changing. I guide and inform you every step of the way to make giving birth abroad part of the adventure rather than a separate event. You will get clear on your choices and you will learn practical tools that work because information is power.

The wireless world knows no boundaries and I am never more than a phone call, text or tweet away. I offer live calls so that we have a relationship in real time. If you want to connect and chat with me personally to explore how I can help you, you will find a link on the website to book a call. If you have not done so already, then head on over and join my Facebook groups and sign up for the gifts on my website www.thevirtualmidwife.com.

I look forward to meeting you on your expat journey and hearing your experiences.

Karen

PS. I would love to know more about you. What drove you to move to another country or did you follow your partner? What are your dreams and aspirations? Please share your experiences on my Facebook page www.facebook.com/thevirtualmidwife.

ABOUT *THE VIRTUAL MIDWIFE*, KAREN WILMOT

Karen qualified in South Africa as a Registered Nurse and Midwife in 1990.

Her career has enabled her to work on a diamond mine in South Africa, in a small village in Mexico, in a military hospital in Saudi Arabia and with the Royal family of Oman. This rich diversity of experience has given her a deep insight into the needs of women across countries and cultures. By stepping out of the hospital labour room, Karen treats birth on the continuum, as the bridge from pregnancy to motherhood. By truly being with women she understands the lifelong impact of the birth experience and how it is bound up with sexuality and parenting. By extending her study of birth outside of her own culture, she learned that in many other cultures it is celebrated and honoured as a rite of passage, with ritual and ceremonies. Karen strives to build a bridge between ancient wisdom and modern knowing.

In 2009 she left the technocratic policy-based hospital system to be able to support women better. She deepened her study to include yoga, breath work and hypnotherapy to provide a more holistic approach that honours the mind-body connection.

Between 2009 and 2015, she established the first private community service in Oman supporting expat women during pregnancy and birth. In 2016, she was instrumental in opening the first centre for Mother and Baby wellness in the Gulf region. She continues to be a pioneer for women's healthcare in the Middle East while developing a programme designed to embrace the uniqueness of every woman.

Her challenge is to develop the discerning and critical use of online technology by teaching strategies, skills and systems that facilitate the principles of adult learning in antenatal education. Her dream is for every woman to give birth with confidence, trust and love.

Acknowledgements

This book would not have been born without the support of Shona MacAngus-Plumridge who I supported eight years ago when her daughter was born. While we had not kept in touch after her birth, we found ourselves sitting next to each other in the hair dresser, both with tufts of foil that kept us immobilised for over an hour as we waited for our highlights to "cure". We reconnected on a deep soul level as we shared the events of the past years and made arrangements to meet up and chat more.

It was during one of those visits that I casually mentioned I was writing a book and attending a conference in Amsterdam. Both of these were true, but I had been writing the book for over three years and in my mind that was enough. I did not think I would ever finish it. Shona did and her absolute belief in me never wavered as she encouraged me to get it done before the conference. With only six weeks to go, she gently guided, coached and encouraged me with regular emails, calls and tons of encouragement.

I finished the first draft one week before I arrived in Amsterdam, giving me enough time to have five proof copies waiting for me at my hotel when I arrived. The feeling of holding my book in my hands was indescribable. I needed another eight months and several revisions for the copy that you are now holding to become available, but it would never have happened without the absolute love and support of Shona. She had absolute faith in me and she pushed me beyond my own limiting beliefs. For that I will be forever grateful.

To the hundreds of families that I have supported over the last 10 years, mainly in Oman and the Middle East, thank you. Each one of you taught me something about myself and my art. The beauty of being a midwife is that we never stop learning, and being with you allows me to do that. We share moments of deep vulnerability and I thank you for your trust and faith in me. Many of you have become lifelong friends. You know who you are.

To the Omani families who welcomed me into your country and your homes, I am forever grateful. I feel so privileged to have been given the many opportunities that living in your beautiful country gave me. Thank you to Lujaina and Lamia Al Kharusi who made my dream of opening a centre for mothers and babies come true.

To Judy Edy, the first person to order my book. We studied nursing together in South Africa and have kept in touch over the last 30 years. Thank you for your support and your joyous love of life. Also to Kerry Foley, Audra Murray, Lynn Webb Kaiser and Tracey Gething Fetting. Many happy nursing memories and so much online love and support.

To the families who shared their stories of giving birth abroad and gave me permission to include details of their experiences as pregnant expats. Thank you for your endless trust in me and my mission to change the world one birth at a time.

And to my mother and father - you would be so proud.

www.thevirtualmidwife.com